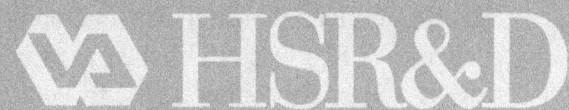

I0470682

Public Presentation of Health System or Facility Data about Quality and Safety: A Systematic Review

October 2011

Prepared for:

Department of Veterans Affairs
Veterans Health Administration
Health Services Research & Development Service
Washington, DC 20420

Prepared by:

Evidence-based Synthesis Program (ESP) Center
West Los Angeles VA Medical Center
Los Angeles, CA
Paul G. Shekelle, M.D., Ph.D., Director

Investigators:

Principal Investigator:
Paul G. Shekelle, M.D., Ph.D.

Co-Investigator:
Isomi M. Miake-Lye, B.A.
Annette M. Totten, Ph.D.
Mary E. Vaiana, Ph.D.

Research Associates:
Jessica M. Beroes, B.S.

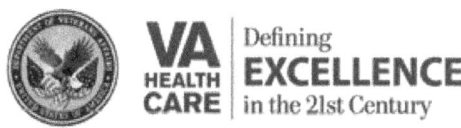

PREFACE

Health Services Research & Development Service's (HSR&D's) Evidence-based Synthesis Program (ESP) was established to provide timely and accurate syntheses of targeted healthcare topics of particular importance to Veterans Affairs (VA) managers and policymakers, as they work to improve the health and healthcare of Veterans. The ESP disseminates these reports throughout VA.

HSR&D provides funding for four ESP Centers and each Center has an active VA affiliation. The ESP Centers generate evidence syntheses on important clinical practice topics, and these reports help:

- develop clinical policies informed by evidence,
- guide the implementation of effective services to improve patient outcomes and to support VA clinical practice guidelines and performance measures, and
- set the direction for future research to address gaps in clinical knowledge.

In 2009, the ESP Coordinating Center was created to expand the capacity of HSR&D Central Office and the four ESP sites by developing and maintaining program processes. In addition, the Center established a Steering Committee comprised of HSR&D field-based investigators, VA Patient Care Services, Office of Quality and Performance, and Veterans Integrated Service Networks (VISN) Clinical Management Officers. The Steering Committee provides program oversight, guides strategic planning, coordinates dissemination activities, and develops collaborations with VA leadership to identify new ESP topics of importance to Veterans and the VA healthcare system.

Comments on this evidence report are welcome and can be sent to Nicole Floyd, ESP Coordinating Center Program Manager, at nicole.floyd@va.gov.

Recommended citation: Totten AM, Miake-Lye IM, Vaiana ME, Beroes JM, Shekelle PG. Public Presentation of Health System or Facility Data about Quality and Safety: A Systematic Review. VA-ESP Project #05-226; 2011

TABLE OF CONTENTS

TABLES

FIGURES

EXECUTIVE SUMMARY

BACKGROUND

The public presentation of quality and safety data is essential to the Department of Veterans Affairs (VA) commitment to transparency. By making data available VA hopes to engage veterans and families in care, promote informed choice, and stimulate performance improvement activities.

The objectives of this project are: 1) to update a recent systematic review of the evidence that making performance data publically available leads to improvements in quality of care and safety; and 2) to summarize current research about patients' and families' use of performance data and how the presentation and distribution of these data could be designed to maximize their use by veterans and family members.

The Key Questions were:

1. What is the most effective way of displaying quality and service information so that it is understandable?
2. How do patients prefer to receive or access this information?
3. What is the evidence that patients or their families use publicly reported quality and safety information to make informed health care decisions?
4. What is the evidence that public reporting of quality and safety information leads to improved quality of safety?

METHODS

We searched Web of Science through 2010 using standard search terms. We limited the search to peer-reviewed articles published in the English language. Additional citations were identified from reference mining and content experts. Titles, abstracts, and articles were reviewed in duplicate by reviewers trained in the critical analysis of literature. All data were narratively summarized.

Study characteristics and key findings were extracted by trained research associates under the supervision of the Principal Investigator. We assessed study quality according to criteria developed by Fung and colleagues, and used AMSTAR grading criteria for systematic reviews.

DATA SYNTHESIS

We constructed evidence tables showing study objective, subject of public reporting, whether the article discusses public reporting of hospital or health plan data, location, sample, study design, key findings and ratings, organized by key question. We analyzed studies to compare their characteristics, methods, and findings. We compiled a summary of findings for each question based on qualitative synthesis of the findings.

PEER REVIEW

A draft version of this report was reviewed by seven technical experts, as well as by clinical leadership. Reviewer comments were addressed and our responses were incorporated in the final report.

RESULTS

We screened 370 titles and rejected 261, and performed a more detailed review on 117 articles. From these, we identified 55 articles that addressed one of the key questions.

Key Questions #1 and #2

We identified reports commissioned by AHRQ and the Robert Wood Johnson Foundation regarding how to best produce and disseminate public reports. Their conclusions about solutions for the design of public reports are three-fold. To make the information more relevant to what consumers already understand and care about, public reports should give an overall definition of quality, define the elements of quality and use them as the reporting categories, and include information about the sponsor and methods. To make it easy for consumers to understand and use the comparative information summarize, interpret, highlight meaning, narrow options and help bring the information together in a choice by using summary measures and meaningful symbols. Finally, testing reports with consumers during development will help identify areas of misunderstanding and assess users' perceptions of the report's value.

Key Question #3

Conclusions from the studies of public reporting are mixed, but most studies found the use of publicly available data to be modest at best. Although consumers may show interest in public reports, in most cases interest does not seem to translate into actual use. The studies that do show use suggest that consumers may avoid low performers, but higher performers may not reap comparable positive benefits of public reporting.

Key Question #4

We identified relatively few new studies within our scope in the peer reviewed literature during the five years since the search was conducted for Fung et al. Two of the newly identified studies addressed the impact of reporting on quality improvement activities. Some empirical evidence and the conclusion of the prior review support the theory that public reporting stimulates quality improvement activities. Five new studies identified address a variety of outcomes (patient or consumer experience, obtaining performance targets, rates of caesarean and mortality) and four of the five are national studies. All five conclude that public reporting has a positive impact on quality or safety outcomes; however, the effect was small and two studies were time series studies in a single country, where all providers were subject to public reporting and the change, each could have been due to other changes that impacted all providers.

This small and varied amount of additional evidence is not sufficient to change the conclusion of the Fung et al. review that "the effect of public reporting on effectiveness, safety, and patient-centeredness remains uncertain." However, the CHOP assessment from 2005 provides some encouragement that this may be changing.

EVIDENCE REPORT

INTRODUCTION

BACKGROUND

The Department of Veterans Affairs (VA) "Open Government Plan" outlines the agency's commitment to transparency, and defines transparency as both increasing access to public information and enabling better engagement and advocacy on behalf of Veterans.[1] Key elements of the transparency initiative involve public presentation of health system and facility data about quality of care and safety. Examples include the VA Hospital Compare website, which provides outcomes and process data for selected diagnoses and the ASPIRE dashboard, which reports quality and safety goals for all VA hospitals.[2]

There are many reasons to make quality and safety information available to the public. One of the key goals of public reporting is to improve the quality of services. Theories and experience suggest multiple pathways from public reporting to health services improvement and ultimately to better patient outcomes. In a situation where patients and families have a choice among health care providers (systems or facilities), quality information makes it possible for patients to select providers based on performance. Public reporting also "levels the playing field" by making the knowledge about quality more accessible to patients. Without public reporting this information may only be known by providers. In turn, concern about loss of market share may motivate providers to improve processes and strive to improve outcomes.[3]

Publicly available data may also give provider organizations direct incentives to improve care. Report cards, rankings, and websites about quality allow organizations to compare their performance to that of their peers, but also make providers aware that others can make these comparisons as well. Concern about reputation can itself be a powerful motivator for change.[4] Patient advocates, policy makers, and the media can also use publicly reported data to identify high and low performing organizations, track change over time, and promote high quality care.

VA is committed to making its publicly reported performance data as accessible and useful as possible. This review and synthesis seeks to identify the key lessons for VA drawn from available research on public reporting that could be applied to future VA transparency efforts.

METHODS

TOPIC DEVELOPMENT

This project was nominated by the Transparency Initiative Lead in the Office of Quality and Performance, Maris Norwood.

The final key questions are:

Key Question #1. What is known about the most effective way of displaying quality and safety information, comparative data about health system structure, services, and performance so that it is understandable?

Key Question #2. How do patients prefer to receive or access this information?

Key Question #3. What is the evidence that patients or their families use publicly reported quality and safety information to make informed health care decisions?

Key Question #4. What is the evidence that public reporting of quality and safety information leads to improved quality or safety?

SEARCH STRATEGY

The topic of public reporting has been reviewed several times, most recently published in 2008 by Fung and colleagues with a literature review current through 2006. We used science citation searches of high-profile reviews and seminal articles as our means to identify new material, in addition to the existing material in the most recent review by Fung and colleagues (Appendix A). We searched Web of Science, with the sub-databases Science (SCI-EXPANDED), Social Science (SSCI), Arts and Humanities (A&HCI), and the Science and Social Sciences Proceedings (CPCI-S C CPCI-SSH) using standard search terms. We searched from the original publication date of the high profile review on seminal articles through July 2011. We chose to keep the publication date criteria open-ended, so no start date was set. We limited the search to articles published in English since we judged that for these key questions, context mattered; for the first two questions, we restricted the articles to those presenting data on English-speaking countries. We also conducted a web search by entering the terms "public reporting of quality information healthcare" into Google and taking the top 30 hits.

STUDY SELECTION

Two reviewers assessed for relevance the abstracts of citations identified from literature searches. Full-text articles of potentially relevant abstracts were retrieved for further review. Each article was reviewed using the eligibility criteria in Appendix B.

Specific exclusion criteria were as follows:

1. Because VA is only anticipating public reporting for facilities, we excluded studies regarding quality and safety information about nursing homes, physicians or other individual providers

2. No key question addressed, or serving background purposes only
3. Non-systematic review, commentary or news, other article with no original data

DATA ABSTRACTION

We abstracted the following data for each included study: study objective, subject of public reporting, whether the article discusses public reporting of hospital or health plan data, location, sample, study design, design rating, key findings, and global rating. (All of the data appear in the evidence tables in Appendix C-E)

QUALITY ASSESSMENT

We assessed the quality of all included studies using criteria developed by Fung and colleagues in order to facilitate the synthesis of results.[5] We replicated the criteria used in this review to evaluate study design and assign global rating. The criteria ranked study design based on four categories, with four stars indicating the strongest design (in general randomized or experimental studies), and one star representing the weakest. The global rating system was modeled after the Grading of Recommendations, Assessment, Development, and Evaluation (GRADE)system,[6] and studies were ranked on whether they should carry great (highest score: 3), moderate (2), or little (1) weight when considering the strength of evidence. The global score takes the study design ranking into account, as well as "penetration of report card use (adherence), dose-response gradient, precision and validity of outcomes, and uncertainty about direction of the results." Systematic reviews were assessed using the AMSTAR grading criteria[7] (see Appendix F for details of all criteria).

DATA SYNTHESIS

We constructed evidence tables showing the study characteristics and results for all included studies, organized by key question. We analyzed studies to compare their characteristics, methods, and findings. We summarized findings for each key question and drew conclusions based on qualitative synthesis of the findings.

PEER REVIEW

A draft version of this report was reviewed by seven technical experts as well as clinical leadership. Their comments and our responses are presented in Appendix G.

RESULTS

LITERATURE FLOW

We reviewed 370 titles and abstracts from the electronic search, one additional reference from reference mining, and 7 others from content experts, for a total of 378. After eliminating clearly irrelevant titles and abstracts, we had 117 references. We retrieved full-text of these articles for further review, and subsequently excluded 97 additional references. We identified a total of 18 references for inclusion in the current review to add to the 37 previously identified in the review by Fung and colleagues. We then grouped the studies by key question. Figure 1 details the exclusion criteria and the number of references related to each of the key questions.

From the Google search of "public reporting of quality information healthcare" (accessed on September 27, 2011) we took the top 30 hits. These were categorized as: websites of organizations that do public reporting, scholarly reports of public reporting (potentially eligible for this review), and other miscellaneous public reporting–related sites. The table lists the 30 hits and their classification.

Table 1. Results from the Google Search

Google Results	Websites or Tools	Scholarly Articles*	Misc.
1. "Dying to Know: Public Release of Information About Quality of Health Care" Marshall, 2000.		Same material as Marshall JAMA 2000 paper	
2. "Best Practices in Public Reporting No. 1" Hibbard, 2010		Included	
3. "Transparency and Public Reporting Are Essential for a Safe Health Care System" Leape, 2010		No original data	
4. "AF4Q areas of focus: Increasing public reporting" RWJF	X		
5. "Putting the Public Back in Public Reporting of Health Care Quality" Lagu, 2010.		No original data	
6. "Public Reporting on Health Care Quality: A Symposium on the "State" of the Art, on June 6, 2006" California Office of the Patient Advocate	X		
7. HCAHPS: http://www.hcahpsonline.org	X		
8. "Hospital Quality Initiatives Overview" Centers for Medicare and Medicaid Services	X		
9. "Healthcare Infection Control Practices Advisory Committee (HICPAC)" Centers for Disease Control and Prevention			X
10. "Public Reporting Key to Cost/Quality Improvements in Health Care" Group Insurance Commission Newsletter, 2009			X
11. "Health Report Cards" Wikipedia			X

Google Results	Websites or Tools	Scholarly Articles*	Misc.
12. "How do we maximize the impact of the public reporting of quality of care?" Marshall, 2004		Included	
13. "Mandatory Reporting of Healthcare Performance Measures" Association for Professionals in Infection Control and Epidemiology	X		
14. "Public Reporting Improves Healthcare" Chen, 2010		No original data	
15. "Public reporting in health care: how do consumers use quality-of-care information? A systematic review. Faber, 2009		Included	
16. Iowa Healthcare Collaborative www.ihconline.org	X		
17. National Quality Forum www.qualityforum.org	X		
18. "Report to Congress: National Strategy for Quality Improvement in Health Care" www.healthcare.gov/law/resources/reports/quality03212011a.html	X		
19. Hospital Compare www.hospitalcompare.hhs.gov	X		
20. Colorado Foundation for Medical Care www.cfmc.org/hospital/hospital_compare.htm			X
21. "Public Reporting of Hospital Quality Indicators" OU Medical Center			X
22. "A Greater Degree of Public Reporting" Marshall, 2002		No original data	
23. "Public Reporting on Health Care Quality" contract bidding with California Office of the Patient Advocate			X
24. "Best Practices in Public Reporting No. 2" Hibbard, 2010		Included	
25. "Essential Tool Kit" CDC	X		
26. "Public reporting of health quality information" Health Affairs Prologue, 2003			X
27. "Crossing the Quality Chasm: The IOM Health Care Quality Initiative" IOM	X		
28. "Public Reporting of Quality Information on Medicaid Health Plans" Felt-Lisk et al., 2007		No KQ addressed	
29. "Health-Care Reform Rules Would Restrict Public Reporting" ProPublica		News article	
30. "Public reporting of comparative information about quality of healthcare" Marshall, 2002		No original data	

* Exclusion criteria given for articles not in this review

All scholarly articles marked as includes in the table were identified and included in our report, and thus already recorded in our flow (Figure 1).

Figure 1. Literature Flow

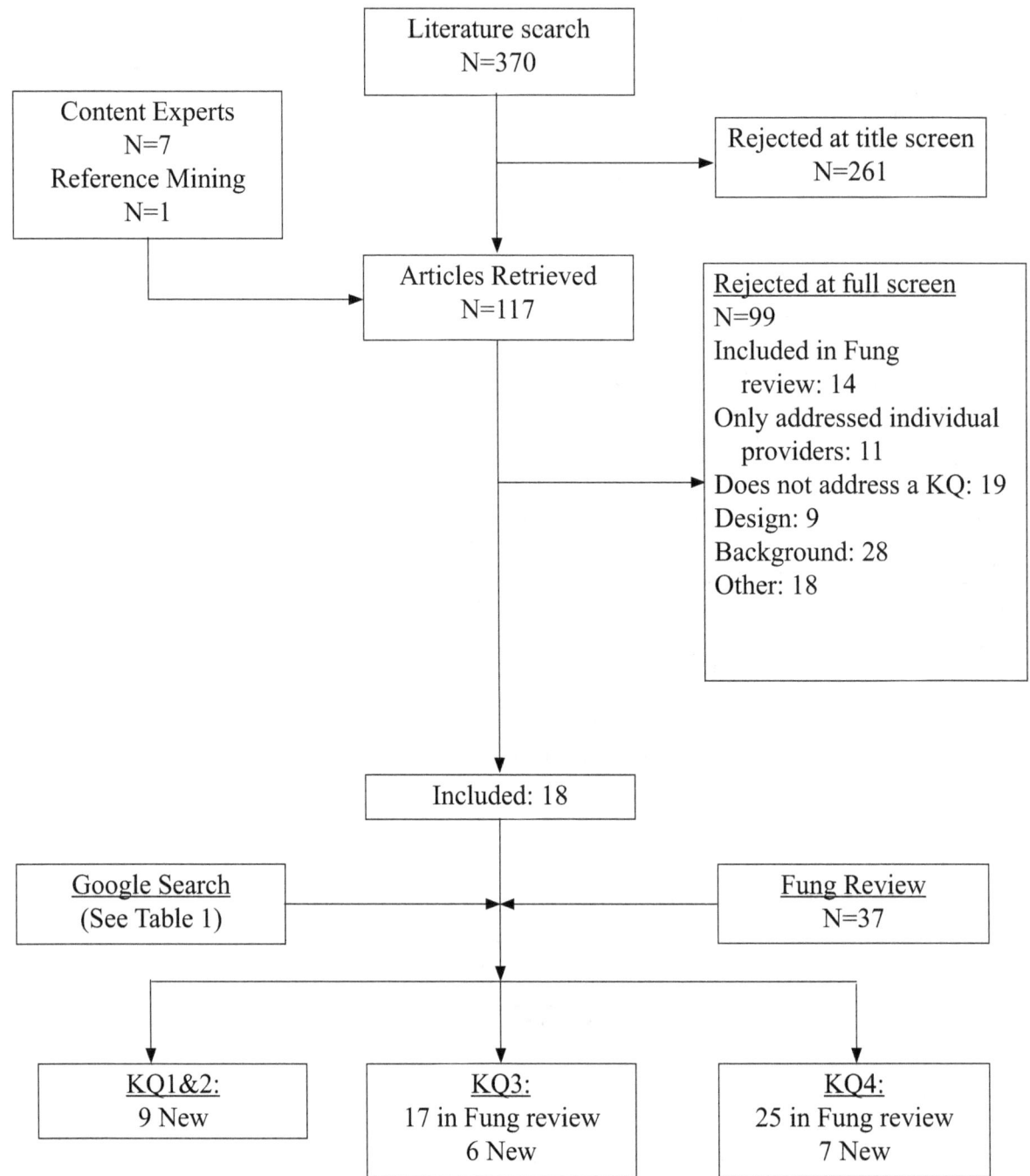

Prior Reviews

This report is the third in a series of systematic reviews with a similar focus on the effects of public reporting on performance. The 2008 systematic review by Fung and colleagues served as a foundation for the current report's search strategies and evidence base.[5] However, their scope was slightly different: they were examining how publishing performance data improves quality of care—in particular, they included individual provider data, which we do not include here.

Fung et al. identified 45 articles evaluating the impact of public reporting on quality-- 10 studies focused on public reporting of health plan data, 27 focused on hospital data, and 11 focused on individual provider data. These categories were not mutually exclusive, but we include only those articles examining public reporting of health plans or hospitals in the present report. They categorized their data in two steps. First, articles were categorized by the level of data: health plan, hospital, or individual providers. Then they were categorized by outcome: whether the public reporting targeted the selection pathway for improving performance, influenced quality improvement activity, affected clinical outcomes, or had unintended consequences (see Figure 2).

Figure 2. Two pathways for improving performance through release of publicly reported performance data[3]

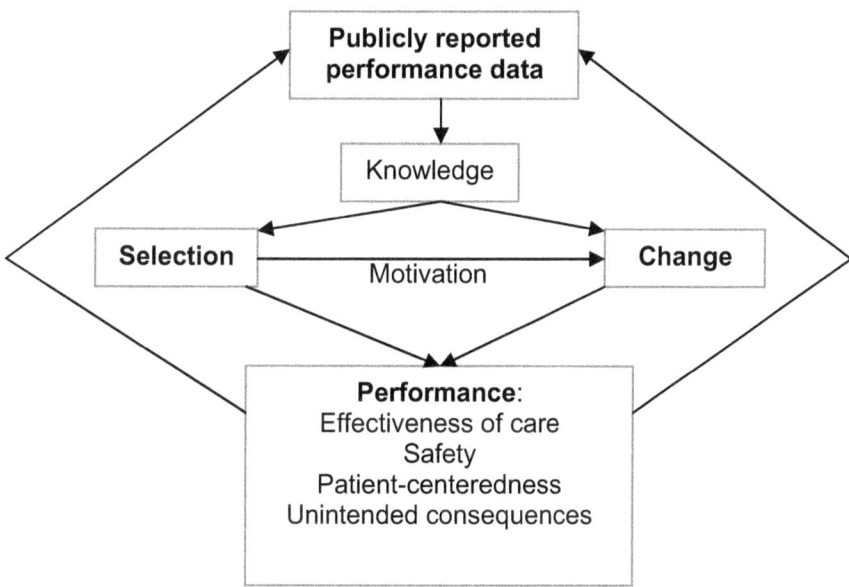

Fung et al. found an overall scarcity of data. However, the existing data suggested that public reporting stimulates quality improvement activity at the hospital level. In the other contexts examined (health plans, individual providers) and for other outcomes, its effects could not be stated with certainty.

An earlier review was published by Marshall and colleagues.[8] They identified a total of 21 peer-reviewed publications, which reported studies of seven public reporting systems. They sought to answer two key questions: (1) Who uses public reports (consumers, purchasers, physicians, hospitals and other provider organizations); and (2) What is the impact of public reporting on quality of care outcomes and costs.

In response to the first question, Marshall et al. found that hospitals and other provider organizations appear to be the most responsive to publicly reported data, leading them to conclude that this pathway may be the most productive area for future research. They reported that consumers, purchasers, and physicians did not understand or trust performance data; these groups made only modest use of the data and public reporting had only slight effects on them. The limited number of studies they found addressing the second question supported an association between public reporting and improvements in health outcomes.

Reporting Systems That Have Been the Subject of Published Evaluations

Like the Marshall and Fung reviews, we found that a relatively small number of reporting systems have been evaluated (see Figure 3). Of the 47 articles we identified that evaluated a particular public reporting system, 15 concerned the New York State Cardiac Surgery Reporting System (CSRS), and another 7 concerned the Consumer Assessment of Health Plans (CAHPS) and 5 concerned the Cleveland Health Quality Choice program (CHQC). Thus these three public reporting systems account for more than half of the published evaluations. Yet a recent environmental scan of public reporting systems performed by Mathematica for the National Quality Forum identified 70 public reporting programs in the US.[9] Consequently, we conclude that most US public reporting systems are not the subject of evaluation or research described in the peer reviewed literature.

Figure 3. Reporting Systems Represented

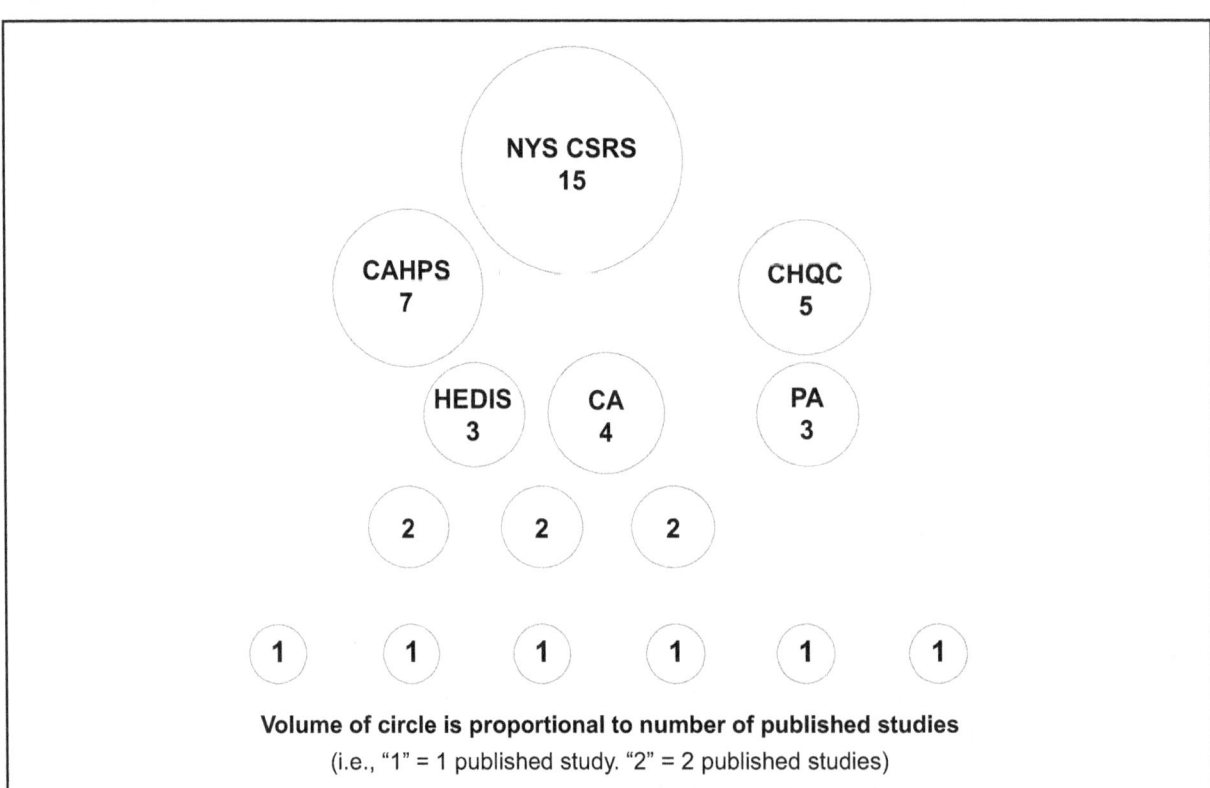

NYS CSRS=New York State Cardiac Surgery Reporting System; CAHPS=Consumer Assessment of Health Plans; CHQC= Cleveland Health Quality Choice program; HEDIS= Healthcare Effectiveness Data and Information Set; CA= Public reporting systems in California, including the California Hospital Outcomes Project (CHOP); PA=Pennsylvania public reporting system.
Two mentions: Federal Employee Health Benefit guide; QualityCounts; public reporting from the UK, including the National Health Service (NHS).
One mention: Health Care Financing Administration (HCFA); Buyers Health Care Action Group (BHCA); Institute for Clinical Evaluative Sciences (ICES) Ontario; Missouri Department of Health's obstetrics consumer report; Dutch national survey of consumer experience measures (based on CAHPS); national caesarean rates in South Korean hospitals

KEY QUESTIONS #1 AND #2. What is known about the most effective way of displaying quality and safety information, comparative data about health system structure, services, and performance so that it is understandable? How do patients prefer to receive or access this information?

We identified two major sources of information about effective ways to report comparative quality information to health care consumers. The first, *Best Practices in Public Reporting*,[10-12] is a recent series of reports that directly address the issue of how to present information to consumers. The series is part of the Learning Network tool set developed by the Agency for Healthcare Research and Quality.[13] The tool set is intended to provide practical approaches to designing public reports that make health care performance information clear, meaningful, and usable by consumers, who may have limited time or motivation to access such information. While these reports are not systematic reviews per se, they were commissioned by AHRQ and written by leading authorities in the field and intended to present both empirical and experiential evidence specific to these two key questions.

The audiences for the reports include Chartered Value Exchanges and other community collaboratives. The reports, which provide general guidelines for presenting information, are intended for use by States, health plans, and purchasers involved in producing, packaging, promoting, and disseminating comparative health care quality and cost information for consumers, patients, and the general public.

The second major source is the *Aligning Forces for Quality (AF4Q)* initiative—the signature effort of the Robert Wood Johnson Foundation to improve the quality of health care in targeted communities.[14, 15] AF4Q operates in 17 regions nationwide, with the goal of bringing together everyone who gets, gives, and pays for health care to improve the quality of care provided locally and to provide models for national reform.[16] The AF4Q documents present general guidelines for reporting information in user friendly ways. In addition, they provide more focused guidelines for reporting specific kinds of information or reporting to specific audiences—for example, *Language to Use in Public Reporting About Hospital Care*,[17] *How to Describe the Health and Community Context for Comparative Performance Reports*,[18] and *Communicating with Physicians about Performance Measurement*.[19]

In addition to these two major sources, six other studies were also identified in the search used to update the Fung et al. review. Four are discussed below as they relate to the findings of the *Best Practices in Public Reporting* and the *Aligning Forces for Quality*.[20-23] The final two are from the Andalusian Health Service[24] and the German national hospital system;[25] we did not include them in our synthesis because we restricted the evidence for these two questions to US data, since the findings are particularly sensitive to context.

How to Effectively Present Health Care Performance Data to Consumers

In this report, for the most part we will use the term, "consumers" and "patients" interchangeably, although "patients" may be construed as Veterans while "consumers" is a commonly used term in discussions of public reporting and includes patients and others, such as family members, who make health care decisions.

Giving consumers comparative performance information is part of an overall strategy to improve health care. Performance reporting has two basic underlying assumptions:

- Consumers will use performance information to choose high-quality health care for themselves and their family members.

- Consumer choices will collectively stimulate quality improvement among providers seeking to protect or improve their market share, or to protect or enhance their public reputations.

Designers of performance "report cards" face four major challenges:[10, 11]

1. **Consumers are not interested in report cards**: they believe care is high quality and uniform across providers.
2. **Consumers and clinical experts define quality differently**. Performance reports include both technical quality of care measures and patient experience measures. Consumers identify the latter, but not the former, as critical components of quality care.
3. **Quality measures are often hard to understand or are not meaningful to consumers**. For example, hospital performance reports may use length of stay as an indicator of poor performance. But consumers may think longer length of stay indicates high quality—e.g., patients can stay as long as they need to get well. Other measures don't make sense to consumers—e.g., administration of beta blockers and angiotensin-converting enzyme (ACE) inhibitors. What consumers don't understand they ignore.
4. **Using quality information to inform choices is hard**. Using a performance report to choose a provider requires consumers to process a great deal of information, identify the factors that they care about and weight them accordingly, and integrate all the factors into a choice. This process requires comparatively high level analytical skills and places a substantial cognitive burden on the users of public reports. Most people lack related skills and experiences.

Two articles identified in our searches support these findings.[20, 22] Mazor and colleagues report that patients choosing a hospital are more likely to rely on factors such as the prior experience of the consumer (95%), reputation of the hospital (93%), physician recommendation (92%), and insurance coverage (91%) than they are to use safe practice score (82%), infection rates (82%), and mortality rates (76%).[20] Another study found that participants were most interested in having cardiac report cards provide information about the experiences of other cardiac patients.[22]

Practical Solutions for Designing Reports

Hibbard and Sofaer (2010)[10] suggest multiple strategies for designing performance reports that consumers can, and will, actually use.

1. Make the information in the report relevant to what consumers already understand.

> An overall **definition of quality, couched in everyday language**—for example, "care that does not cause harm"—can help consumers develop a broader view of quality. Using the **components of the definition as the reporting categories** can help consumers link the ratings to things they care about. Consumers also know that their own personal experiences with care vary. The hope

is that "pairing information on the technical aspects of quality with patient experience data" will alert consumers to the importance of understanding what quality of care means.

As in other areas, consumers prefer to have information from a trusted source. This means that reports should **include information about who sponsored the report, how the information was gathered, and where additional details can be found**.

2. *Make it easier for consumers to understand and use the information.*

Key techniques are **summarizing and interpreting the data and highlighting meaning**— for example, by labeling performance as "excellent" or "poor" or ranking ordering providers by performance. Cognitive signposts such as "best value" can help consumers to digest evaluations of multiple factors. Since about one-half of the population finds it difficult to interpret numbers, using **symbols can be helpful**—especially if the symbol conveys the meaning directly and helps consumers to identify a pattern. An example would be combining the word "below" with a downward pointing triangle.

Such strategies help report users to bring diverse information together in a choice. The capabilities of the Web can be exploited to **help consumers filter and customize information.** Hibbard and Sofaer provide examples of these strategies, noting that strategies most helpful to consumers are often ones that providers resist—e.g., ordering providers by some specific, or summary, dimension of performance.

3. *Test the report with consumers to learn what does and doesn't work.*

Key techniques include asking individuals to explain in their own words what a label or symbol means. Giving users "assignments" such as finding the top three or bottom three performers reveals whether the information in the report is presented in a way that supports a choice. A recent experiment identified report features that consumers found most helpful:[23] ordering by level of performance rather than alphabetical order, using meaningful symbols instead of numbers, providing an overall summary measure, and including fewer reporting categories.

Table 2 summarizes the practical design suggestions offered by Hibbard and Sofaer.

Table 2. Summary of Design Solutions for Performance Reports

Make the information more relevant to what consumers already understand and care about
<ul><li>Give an overall definition of quality</li><li>Define the elements of quality and use them as the reporting categories</li><li>Include information about the sponsor and methods</li></ul>
Make it easy for consumers to understand and use the comparative information
<ul><li>Summarize, interpret, highlight meaning, narrow options</li><li>Help to bring the information together in a choice by using summary measures and meaningful symbols</li></ul>
Test reports with consumers during development
<ul><li>Identify areas of misunderstanding</li><li>Assess users' perceptions of the report's value</li></ul>

Mazor and colleagues found no statistical difference in consumers' ability to interpret the content of reports when key elements of how the information was presented were changed: consistency of hospital performance across indicators, presentation type, or presence of confidence intervals.[20] Despite these variations, consumers were able to correctly interpret the data, with a "vast majority" of respondents correctly identifying hospitals with the best safety or infection scores. In another study by Mazor and colleagues, actual numerical scores and print reports, as opposed to symbols and online reports, were preferred in 59 qualitative interviews discussing consumer views of public reports on Health Care-Associated Infections.[21]

The *AF4Q* reports address the same display challenges but couch them as display goals, along with display strategies to achieve them.[14, 15] Table 3 summarizes the goals and strategies.

Table 3. Goals of a Good Display of Comparative Information

Strategy	Goal Achieved		
	Makes it easier to identify and understand patterns	Helps users focus on topics or providers of interest	Reduces amount of information for users
Explicit points of comparison	X		
Symbols	X		
Word icons	X		
Helping users limit the number of providers	X	X	
Rank ordering and tiering	X	X	
Quality framework	X	X	
Composite measures		X	X
Summary scores			X

The *AF4Q* reports provide guidance about how to implement each of these strategies and give "before" and "after" illustrations to demonstrate how the strategy may be applied.[14, 15]

Cost and Efficiency

Increasingly, cost data are being included in public performance reports. These data are often misinterpreted, especially since Americans tend to think that higher cost always translates to higher quality. Showing quality within cost strata or cost within quality strata may demonstrate that high quality care isn't necessarily the most expensive care.

Consumers are not accustomed to thinking about the efficiency of health care, and they may equate efficiency with cutting corners or saving money for their employer. Hibbard and Sofaer suggest some terminology that might help to clarify the concept of efficiency—e.g., "Uses health care dollars wisely"—but suggest additional testing is needed to determine what works best for consumers.[10]

Maximizing Consumer Understanding of Public Comparative Quality Reports: Effective Use of Explanatory Information

Having a set of provider performance measures and ratings does not make an effective public report. Sofaer and Hibbard (2010)[11] identify explanatory information needed to accurately communicate quality ratings to consumers and motivate them to use the information to inform their health care decisions.

The report offers nine evidence-based recommendations and related examples:

1. *Engage and motivate consumers to explore and use reports*.
    The first page of a report, whether in hard copy or online, should **include key messages** to motivate the user. For example, "A poor choice of provider can have serious consequences for your health and finances."

2. *Deepen consumers' understanding of health care quality and quality measures*.
    Provide a broad framework that defines different aspects of quality and helps consumers link what they care about to the more sophisticated quality measures presented in the report. **Clearly state the purpose and value** of the report.

3. *Legitimize the report's sponsor and the report's credibility*.
    Consumers want to know **who is issuing the report and why**, whether the report's ratings are fair, and how the performance scores were generated. Technical details should be accessible but most consumers won't consult them.

4. *Provide information about the importance, meaning, and interpretation of specific measures*.
    Measures should be described and interpreted in everyday language; different types of measures—e.g., patient experience measures versus outcome measures such as patient safety or mortality—will need to be explained. Consumers may need **guidance about what to look for in a graph**.

5. *Help consumers understand the implications of resource use information*.
    The term **"resource use" has not been tested with consumers**, so it is not clear how they interpret it. Two general beliefs are barriers to appropriate interpretation: the belief that more care is better, and the belief that cost reflects quality.

6. *Help consumers avoid common pitfalls that lead to misinterpretation of quality data*.
    Consumers need to understand that providers should not be compared on certain measures—e.g., very rare events, and that a provider's **overall performance can't be assessed from a limited set of measures** that reflect only part of the provider's services.

7. *Provide consumers guidance and support in using the information*.
    Approaches to providing decision support include **giving consumers a list of what they should think about in choosing a health care provider**—for example, does the provider speak a language other than English, how easy is it to make an appointment, is the provider's office conveniently located for the consumer. A **label or symbol** can help consumers summarize scores—for example, "Best Value." Key differences in performance can be highlighted. **Stories and testimonials** can demonstrate how health information can be used. Reports should also **inform consumers what they can do to protect themselves** from poor quality care since some report users will not have a choice of providers.

8. *Provide access to more detailed information*.
    Web-based reports make it easier to balance ease of use with access to details since consumers can drill down for more information on topics of special interest.

9. *Test the report with consumers before going live.*
    Cognitive interviews are the gold standard for testing surveys and can help guide
    development and revision of the report.

How to Maximize Public Awareness and Use of Comparative Quality Reports through Effective Promotion and Dissemination Strategies

If consumers do not know about publicly available performance reports, they cannot use
them. As a result, report sponsors will have no return on what is often a substantial investment
in creating the report. Unfortunately, few sponsors have been completely successful in
disseminating information about their reports, whether web-based or print, and little research has
been conducted about how to effectively promote and disseminate performance information.

Drawing on insights from social marketing and web marketing, Sofaer and Hibbard (2010)[12]
suggest 10 ways in which report sponsors can promote public awareness and use of comparative
quality reports.

1. Plan from the outset of the project to promote and disseminate the report. Dissemination
    should not be an afterthought.

2. Identify the main audience as early as possible since the nature of the audience drives many
    other choices. An important secondary audience comprises those who are being rated. They
    should receive the report before it goes public.

3. Engage those who can provide information about the nature of the audience and how best to
    reach them. Consumer and patient advocacy groups can play key roles.

4. Use the insights of social marketing. These include paying careful attention to developing the
    key messages for promoting the report. In general, people respond better to messages telling
    them how to protect themselves than they do to messages about how to find the "best" provider.

5. Be strategic about timing the report's release. Few people will be making a provider choice at
    the time the report appears, so audiences need to be reminded frequently that the report exists
    and how to access it.

6. Be strategic about positioning. Identify the places that the key audience(s) go to find health
    information and the kinds of sites or locations that they are likely to access and trust.

7. Work actively with the media to promote the report. Relationships with the media should
    be built early in the project. Guidelines for interacting with the media will help promote a
    consistent message.

8. Use advertising to promote the report. Advertising can reach both broad and specific
    populations.

9. Use outreach to promote the report and facilitate its use. Work with organizations who have
    an ongoing relationship with your audience(s) to give the report visibility. Public libraries
    also offer possibilities for promoting and disseminating the report.

10. Gather and analyze feedback on the report and its dissemination. Web surveys and focus groups
    are just two ways of gathering feedback, which can help inform future reporting efforts.

KEY QUESTION #3. What is the evidence that patients or their families use publicly reported quality and safety information to make informed health care decisions?

The evidence in this section comes from three sources: the review by Fung and colleagues,[5] a newer review by Faber and colleagues specific to consumer's use of quality of care information,[26] and studies not included in either review (see Table 4) that were identified in our search. Articles already summarized in the prior reviews are not necessarily individually discussed.

Table 4. Key Question #3 Article Overlap

Articles in this section	Fung et al.	Faber et al.	Added in this synthesis
Mazor, 2009[20]*			X
Mazor, 2009[21]*			X
Dixon, 2008[27]			X
Peters, 2007[28]		X	
Jha, 2006[29]	X		
Jin, 2006[30]	X		
Uhrig, 2006[31]		X	
Hibbard, 2005[4]	X		
Richard, 2005[22]*			X
Cutler, 2004[32]			X
Romano, 2004[33]	X		
Baker, 2003[34]	X		
Beaulieu, 2002[35]	X		
Chassin, 2002[36]	X		
Farley, 2002[37]	X	X	
Farley, 2002[38]	X	X	
Harris, 2002[39]	X	X	
Harris, 2002[40]			X
Hibbard, 2002[41]		X	
Hibbard, 2002[42]		X	
Scanlon, 2002[43]	X		
Uhrig, 2002[44]		X	
Wedig, 2002[45]	X		
Hibbard, 2001[46]		X	
Shoenbaum, 2001[47]		X	
Hibbard, 2000[48]		X	
Spranca, 2000[49]	X	X	
Knutson, 1998[50]		X	
Mukamel, 1998[51]	X		
Mennemeyer, 1997[52]	X		
Hibbard, 1996[53]		X	
Hannan, 1994[54]	X		
Vladeck, 1988[55]	X		

Discussion of these three articles is in KQ1 and 2.

Evidence from a Systematic Review by Fung and colleagues

The systematic review by Fung and colleagues addresses key question three in their discussion of selection of health plans and hospitals.[5] This review scored a 10/11 using the AMSTAR grading criteria for systematic reviews (see Appendix F). Within a conceptual framework for quality improvement developed by Berwick and colleagues, selection is one of two pathways in which public reporting can improve performance (See Figure 2, page 9).[3] As opposed to the change pathway, in which providers are both the subjects and consumers of the public reporting, the selection pathway is focused on how patients and their intermediaries use publicly reported data in their decision-making process. Because the scope of the current ESP review excludes individual providers, the most applicable findings from this review are those that address the selection of health plans and hospitals.

Fung and colleagues found eight studies, all published after 1999, that addressed the effects of public reporting on selection of health plans. Two randomized, controlled trials using CAHPS survey data in Medicaid beneficiaries' plan selection found no effect on overall selection.[37, 38] However, the analysis did detect an effect in a subgroup who chose an HMO with dominant market share:[37] The participants who read the report selected higher scoring plans compared with the control group. Another two studies using hypothetical performance ratings found that consumers were willing to accept access restrictions or less generous coverage if included providers had higher quality or ratings.[39, 49]

The other four studies in this section used longitudinal observational data and econometric models. Two found that higher scoring plans were chosen more often by federal employees,[30, 45] though employees overall did not switch plans.[30] Employees of Harvard University were more likely to switch plans if they were enrolled with low scorers, as compared to those in higher-scoring plans.[35] Finally, employees of General Motors were most affected by negative ratings, avoiding below-average plans but showing less discrimination with regards to superior ratings.[43] Taken as a whole, the conclusions of these eight studies are mixed, but suggest that public reporting may have modest impact by encouraging people to avoid lower-ranked plans or weigh the benefits of more restricted, higher quality plans.

Nine studies indicated that, in general, selection of hospitals was not affected by publicly reported performance data. Two articles pre-dating 2000 reported on public reporting systems of the Health Care Financing Administration, now the Centers for Medicare and Medicaid Services. These studies found that the public release of hospital mortality rates had a small but statistically significant impact on utilization,[52] but no statistically significant effect when comparing high- and low- mortality hospital occupancy.[55] Another four studies examined the New York State Cardiac Surgery Reporting System (CSRS). Three studies all found that the NYS CSRS had little to no impact on market share.[29, 36, 54] In contrast, the fourth study by Mukamel and Mushlin found higher market share growth rates for providers with better outcomes when compared to those with worse outcomes.[51] The final three studies on hospital selection contributed to the evidence suggesting that public reporting has, at best, selective and short term effects,[33] or, otherwise, little to no effect at all.[4, 34]

Evidence from a Systematic Review by Faber and Colleagues

In a 2009 systematic review that was specific to consumers' use of quality of care information,

Faber and colleagues found 14 eligible studies.[26] Of these, 10 assessed "laboratory experiments," meaning studies of potential consumers making choices about hypothetical situations. The remaining four studies assessed actual "real world" public reports, and all of these were about CAHPS. Two of these studies were also included in the review by Fung and colleagues, as were two other "laboratory experiment" studies (see Table 3).[37-39, 49] This report also scored 10/11 based on the AMSTAR criteria (see Appendix F). Overall, Faber et al. found that "patients often are unaware of the availability of the quality information."[26] Even if the data are identified, consumers "have difficulties in understanding the information," do not view it as useful, and do not use it in their decision-making process. Studies examining consumer attitudes towards publicly reported data found that consumers were very interested in quality of care information. However, this interest does not translate into actual use. The percentage of consumers who were actually influenced by quality information was extremely low.

Evidence Not Included in Prior Reviews

We identified six studies in our literature search that examined consumer use of public reporting. Three of the studies relate to what factors influence patient use of publicly reported data; these have been discussed in the section for key questions one and two.[20-22]

Dixon and colleagues compared employees in one of three health plan options: a high-deductible consumer-directed health plan (CDHP), a lower deductible CDHP, and a preferred provider organization (PPO).[27] The information-seeking behavior of the three plans varied at the outset, with lower-deductible CDHP enrollees being the most active before enrollment and the high-deductible CDHP enrollees using cost information more than those in the PPO. However, over the course of the study, the variation in information seeking between plans decreased. Given this shift towards uniformity, Dixon et al. note that other factors may be better indicators of information use, including enrollee characteristics.

In a cross-sectional time series study examining the New York State Cardiac Surgery Reporting System, Cutler and colleagues found that hospitals that had been flagged as high-mortality experienced a decline in coronary artery bypass surgery (CABG) cases, with a statistically significant decline in all patients in the first year.[32] In both the first and second years, there was a statistically significant decrease in low severity patients, which suggests that hospitals are not simply declining high severity cases to lower their mortality rates. Hospitals with a low mortality ranking did not see statistically significant changes in their number of cases, which supports the notion that lower quality hospitals are more significantly impacted by public reporting than higher quality hospitals. The authors note that the observed changes could be attributable to multiple factors, and that patient decision making is only one such factor. Other demand-side factors such as referral patterns or supply-side factors such as poorly-rated surgeons exiting the market may also contribute to these findings.

In a complex economic analysis of survey data collected at the time of choice, Harris and colleagues found that some attributes of a report card and the survey can be related to actual plan choice.[40] In other words, the authors offer the conclusion "we find evidence that consumers perceive quality and cost differences across health systems," including such factors as distance to the closest provider, cost of the premium, and access to specialists and waiting times.

Summary of Findings

Conclusions from the studies of public reporting are mixed, but most studies found the use of publicly available data to be modest at best. Although consumers may show interest in public reports, in most cases interest does not seem to translate into actual use. The studies that do show use suggest that consumers may avoid low performers, but higher performers may not reap comparable positive benefits of public reporting.

KEY QUESTION #4. What is the evidence that public reporting of quality and safety information leads to improved quality or safety?

Result of Identified Studies

Fung and colleagues identified two groups of studies relevant to the question of whether public reporting leads to improved quality or safety. The first group addressed the question indirectly by examining the impact of public reporting on quality improvement activities; in the second group the outcomes related to public reporting are clinical changes or unintended consequences that are directly associated with quality and safety.

Impact on Quality Improvement Activity

In our update, we identified two new studies that measured whether public reporting affected the quantity of quality improvement activity at hospitals or other health care organizations.[56, 57] The information about the 11 studies identified in the review by Fung and colleagues in which the quantity of quality improvement was the outcome is reproduced in the evidence tables (see Appendix E).

Wang and colleges,[57] in a National Bureau of Economic Research Working Paper, assessed the effect of a "bad" report card (negative rating) on CABG surgery has on surgical volume for hospitals and surgeons. Only the hospital results are discussed here. No statistically significant overall effect was observed. However, one year after being identified as a high mortality hospital, there was a significantly significant drop in quarterly volume of 15 CABG procedures. This drop was primarily due to a decrease in low severity CABG cases.

All 11 studies from the Fung and colleagues review where the reported outcome was quality improvement activities were studies of hospitals; none were identified for health plans. The studies examined public reports of different health care quality data in several geographic areas.

Two studies of the QualityCounts program by Hibbard and colleagues[4, 58] compared the hospitals that experienced public reporting to those that received confidential feedback (available only to the hospitals, not to the public) and others that received no data. They concluded that quality improvement increased in the areas associated with the indicators in the public reports and that hospitals with more quality improvement activities had higher performance scores. Three studies focused on public reporting of CABG surgery mortality in New York or Pennsylvania.[36, 59, 60] These studies use case series, case studies, and surveys to document that hospitals responded to the public reporting of mortality data by improving programs,[36] changing practice patterns[59] and monitoring performance.[60] Other studies documented implementation of quality improvement in Canadian hospitals following public reporting about care for acute MI;[61] the responses of

Cleveland hospitals to a regional reporting effort;[62] and improvements following the release of the Missouri's Consumer Obstetrics Report Card.[63]

However, not all the identified studies found increases in quality improvement activities. Mannion[64] identified cases in England where public reports discouraged improvement even though they were used by hospitals to tailor programs to national targets. Additionally, two studies of the California Hospital Outcomes Project (CHOP) documented limited impact.[65, 66] In response to a survey, only three of 17 California public hospitals reported adding quality improvement activities due to CHOP.[65] Hospital leaders who were surveyed reported that CHOP did not lead to changes in care for acute myocardial infarction, though some respondents did say they used CHOP to identify potential areas for improvement.

A more recent assessment of CHOP examined the impact of reporting on health plans and medical groups.[56] This evaluation is available in the California office of the patients advocate's website. The study documents increasing use up through the last year data collection, 2004, with 28,000 visitors to the website and 100,000 booklets distributed in that year. Most users are interested in the comparing HMO performance in the "plan of service" domain, which includes items such as how quickly the plan handles complaints, getting patient needed care, and overall rating of service. Competitive information on prevention indicators were used less. Compared to those data from 1988 through 1990, the 2005 assessment found that 47% of medical groups and 13% of health plans were undertaking quality improvement activities in response to CHOP.

Impact on Clinical Outcomes

The second group of studies examines how public reporting affects clinical outcomes, including any unintended consequences. In our update we identified five relevant studies in addition to those included in the prior review. In the text below we first describe the newly identified studies in some detail, then summarize the articles include in the Fung review.

The newly identified articles include three about hospitals,[32, 67, 68] one about health plans[69] and one about ambulance services.[70] All document that public reporting had a positive impact on the outcomes of interest.

The Consumer Assessment of Healthcare Providers and System (CAHPS) project is a US government-funded effort to collect and publicly report standardized survey data on patient experiences. Elliot and colleagues[68] assess changes in response to the hospital version of CAHPS between 2008 and 2009—the first two years the data were publicly available (including 61% and 84% of US hospitals, respectively). They found small improvements (from 0.3 to 0.9%) in the mean percentage of patients selecting the most positive responses on 8 out 9 domains. The largest improvement was in "responsiveness of hospital staff" while no improvement was found in "doctor communication." Though small, the improvements were statistically significant and were sufficient to change a hospital's rank. The authors conclude the results suggest that improvement in these domains is possible and may be furthered by public reporting; however, ongoing analyses will be required to see if improvements continue over multiple years.

Cutler and colleagues[32] added to a large literature on the New York State Cardiac Reporting System (CSRS) by conducting a time series analyses of mortality data from all New York hospitals performing bypass surgery. Their analyses examined changes in each hospital's mortality one year after the mortality rates were made public. They found that identification as a high-mortality hospital was associated with improved future performance. Specifically, the improvement in risk adjusted mortality was a statistically significant 1.2 percentage points lower over the 12 months following public reporting as a high-mortality hospital. This improvement persists for an additional 12 months. No significant improvement was found for hospitals that had low mortality rates at the time of the first report.

Kim and colleagues[67] evaluated the impact of public reporting on caesarean rates at hospitals in South Korea, comparing rates before and after the public release of rates in 2000. Overall rates were 43.0% of all deliveries in 1999; 38.6% in 2000 and 39.6% in 2001. Hospitals that had higher caesarean rates in 1999 or did more deliveries were more likely to reduce rates; other organizational factors such as ownership and market share were not associated with decreases in caesarean rates for these years.

Hendriks[69] and her coauthors report on the performance of Dutch health plans over four years (2005-2008) on consumer experience measures from a Dutch survey based on the CAHPS survey used in the US. Overall, health plans improved in four of seven domains: "general rating," "conduct of employees," "health plan information," and "transparency on payment requirements." In an analysis stratified by 2005 performance, plans scoring below average had larger improvements in 2008 scores than did plans scoring average or above average in 2005, across all seven domains. These changes were statistically significant in all domains except "getting the needed help from the call center." The public reports included the data comparing plans as well as press releases that identified specific areas for improvement; however, improvement was not greater in areas publicly identified as needing attention.

Bevan and Hamblin[70] assessed the impact of public reporting on the performance of ambulance services in Great Britain. All the countries in Great Britain had the same targets for ambulance response times, but only in England was the performance for each service included in published 'star ratings' showing whether services met the targets. The frequency with which services met the time targets for different types of calls were tracked from 2000 through 2005. In England, where performance was publicly reported, the percent of calls meeting the target increased. But the percent meeting the target remained low over the same period in Wales and Scotland; indeed performance would have been scored as failing if the English reporting system has been applied to their performance.

The authors conducted analyses to determine if the improvement in England could be attributed to "gaming" or poor data collection. However, even with adjustments for these factors, the improvement in the English services remained significantly better compared with the countries where performance was not publically reported.

These five additional studies supplement the evidence identified and summarized from 14 studies of hospitals and 2 of health plans by Fung et al. The majority (14 of 16) of the studies of hospitals are about two public reporting systems.

Ten of these studies examined the impact of New York State public reporting of mortality rates for cardiac surgery and percutaneous coronary interventions (PCI). Four studies found that mortality rates decreased after public reporting: in a case study of one hospital (6.6% declined to 1.8%);[59] in all New York hospitals after risk-adjustment (4.17% declined to 2.34%).[71] In New York hospitals for elderly patients, mortality declined at a rate faster than the national trend.[72] After public reporting, mortality rates no longer differed across hospitals that had the highest, middle, and lowest rates before the public reporting program.[54]

Two studies did not find a link between public reporting and improvement. Ghali compared New York rates to Massachusetts, a state without public reporting, and found that the decrease in mortality was similar.[73] A comparison of New York and Michigan found lower unadjusted rates for New York, but the difference was no longer significant when the rates were risk adjusted.[74]

Other studies of the New York public reporting system sought to determine if public reporting had unintended consequences on practice patterns, particularly the selection of patients for procedures. The studies came to different conclusions. One study comparing the case mix of NY and Michigan PCI patients found that high-risk patients in NY were less likely to receive PCI, perhaps because public reporting was encouraging selection of lower risk patients.[74] Another study of mortality rates of New York patients at the Cleveland clinic suggested that the increase in mortality of these out-of-state patients is an indication that sicker patients from New York were referred out of state after public reporting.[75] Dranove and colleague documented shifting of severely ill patients to teaching hospitals in New York and Pennsylvania after these states implemented public reporting .[76] In contrast, the study by Peterson and colleagues looked for but found no evidence that access to coronary artery bypass surgery was restricted for elderly acute MI patients or for high- risk elderly.[72]

Four studies of the Cleveland Health Quality Choice (CHQC) program reported minimal positive impact from public reporting. Risk-adjusted mortality rates for conditions included in CHQC decreased according to one study,[77] but a comparison of Cleveland to the rest of Ohio where there was no public reporting found that declines in mortality rates were similar.[78] An analysis of outlier hospitals with high mortality rates found that they did not improve;[34] a complementary study documented that some decreases in in-hospital mortality were offset by after-discharge mortality, resulting in no decline in 30-day mortality.[79]

The remaining two studies concerned other public reporting systems. The Missouri Department of Health issued a consumer report on obstetrics care and evaluation of outcomes over 5 years (1989 to 1994).[63] The report found that hospitals with high rates of cesarean delivery and hospitals with low rates of vaginal birth after cesarean delivery had statistically significant improvements in performance, and rates of very low birth weight were reduced. Hibbard et al. compared hospitals in Wisconsin that were subject to public reporting to hospitals that received confidential feedback on performance or no data.[4] They found that hospitals whose obstetric performance was low were more likely to improve if there was public reporting, and that public or confidential feedback was associated with improvement.

The review by Fung and colleagues also identified two studies assessing the potential effects of public versus private reporting of quality information. Both studies were retrospective cohorts. Bost found that health plans that voluntarily report performance data outperformed non-publicly reporting health plans,[80] while McCormick and colleagues found that plans with lower quality of care scores were more likely than higher-scoring plans to drop out of public reports.[81]

Summary of Findings

We identified relatively few new studies within our scope in the peer reviewed literature during the five years since the search was conducted for Fung et al. Two of the newly identified studies addressed the impact of reporting on quality improvement activities. Some empirical evidence and the conclusion of the prior review support the theory that public reporting stimulates quality improvement activities. Five new studies identified address a variety of outcomes (patient or consumer experience, obtaining performance targets, rates of caesarean and mortality) and four of the five are national studies. All five conclude that public reporting has a positive impact on quality or safety outcomes; however, the effect was small and two studies were time series studies in a single country, where all providers were subject to public reporting and the change, each could have been due to other changes that impacted all providers.

This small and varied amount of additional evidence is not sufficient to change the conclusion of the Fung et al. review that "the effect of public reporting on effectiveness, safety, and patient-centeredness remains uncertain." However, the CHOP assessment from 2005 provides some encouragement that this may be changing.

Quality of Evidence

For impact on quality improvement activities, only one study compared the number of quality improvement activities across hospitals that did and did not experience public reporting.[58] The rest of the identified studies were case studies, case series, or used surveys or interviews to collect information on use of report cards and volume of quality improvement activities. These studies were rated 1 out 4 for study design and given the lowest global rating.

The studies of clinical outcomes and unintended consequences are more varied in terms of design and their weight in the overall body of evidence (global rating). However, the majority make moderate contributions to the weight of evidence and are time series or designs that include multivariate adjustment (3 out of 4 on the rating of study designs).

SUMMARY AND DISCUSSION

SUMMARY OF EVIDENCE BY KEY QUESTION

Key Questions #1 and #2

We identified reports commissioned by AHRQ and the Robert Wood Johnson Foundation regarding how to best produce and disseminate public reports. Their conclusions about solutions for the design of public reports are three-fold. To make the information more relevant to what consumers already understand and care about, public reports should give an overall definition of quality, define the elements of quality and use them as the reporting categories, and include information about the sponsor and methods. To make it easy for consumers to understand and use the comparative information summarize, interpret, highlight meaning, narrow options and help bring the information together in a choice by using summary measures and meaningful symbols. Finally, testing reports with consumers during development will help identify areas of misunderstanding and assess users' perceptions of the report's value.

Key Question #3

Conclusions from the studies of public reporting are mixed, but most studies found the use of publicly available data to be modest at best. Although consumers may show interest in public reports, in most cases interest does not seem to translate into actual use. The studies that do show use suggest that consumers may avoid low performers, but higher performers may not reap comparable positive benefits of public reporting.

Key Question #4

We identified relatively few new studies within our scope in the peer reviewed literature during the five years since the search was conducted for Fung et al. Two of the newly identified studies addressed the impact of reporting on quality improvement activities. Some empirical evidence and the conclusion of the prior review support the theory that public reporting stimulates quality improvement activities. Five new studies identified address a variety of outcomes (patient or consumer experience, obtaining performance targets, rates of caesarean and mortality) and four of the five are national studies. All five conclude that public reporting has a positive impact on quality or safety outcomes; however, the effect was small and two studies were time series studies in a single country, where all providers were subject to public reporting and the change, each could have been due to other changes that impacted all providers.

This small and varied amount of additional evidence is not sufficient to change the conclusion of the Fung et al. review that "the effect of public reporting on effectiveness, safety, and patient-centeredness remains uncertain." However, the CHOP assessment from 2005 provides some encouragement that this may be changing.

LIMITATIONS

The principal limitation to this review is the limited number of public reporting systems that have been subjected to critical published evaluations. Most of the published evidence about the effects of public reporting concern the Cardiac Surgery Reporting System in New York State (CSRS), the Consumer Assessment of Health Plans (CAHPS), and the Cleveland Health Quality Choice program (CHQC), which was abandoned after five years. Far more public reporting programs in America have not been evaluated compared with those that have. Findings from evaluations that have been conducted should be generalized very cautiously, if at all. There is also the possibility of publication bias: additional evaluations may have been conducted but the results are not easily available in the published, peer-viewed literature. Possible reasons include negative findings, the researcher never submitted findings to a journal due to lack of time/interest, and/or work was completed for a stakeholder who was not interested in journal publications. Other potentially relevant evaluations and studies probably exist, but cannot be identified and synthesized based on an examination of databases that are easily searchable. For example, entering "public reporting of quality information" into Google produces over 19,000,000 hits, a number that is impractical to review. Even using limited search terms produces tens of thousands of hits. We did incorporate a limited Google search, but did not identify any new studies in the top 30 hits.

CONCLUSIONS

Even with these limitations, the evidence is consistent that most consumers do not know about or make little use of publicly available performance data when selecting health services providers. Attention to the summary point of designing performance reports and presentation and dissemination may more fully engage consumers. Yet, even without evidence that public reporting has had much effect via the "selection" pathway, evidence (albeit mixed) suggests that public reporting can still achieve some improvements in processes and outcomes of care by stimulating providers to change. In addition, public reporting furthers the VA's goal of transparency.

Applicability of Findings to the VA Population

None of the evidence we identified studied VA public reporting systems or assessed Veterans' use of non-VA public reporting systems. Nevertheless, it is unlikely that most veterans currently use publicly available data on quality and safety in making choices. Experience from non-VA studies suggests the main way that public reporting improves quality and safety is by motivating individuals and organizations to change care delivery. The mechanisms for this motivation can be varied but seem to include both the desire to attract and maintain patients and the desire to be viewed positively by peers. Whether this same motivation holds true in a system such as the VA, which for many patients is a safety-net provider, is unknown. For veterans who do have a choice in health care providers, presenting VA and non-VA information in the same place and making it similar in content and format will be necessary in order to avoid making the cognitive burden of synthesizing the information too high such that it will not be used by veterans. It is not clear whether public reporting would stimulate future changes in a system such as the VA with a robust quality assessment and feedback system already in place.

RECOMMENDATIONS FOR FUTURE RESEARCH

As VA pursues its transparency goals and continues to expand the quality and safety information made available to Veterans and other stakeholders, there is an opportunity to increase the impact of public reporting on the wellbeing of veterans and to contribute to the knowledge related to public reporting and quality improvement in health care.

Examples of specific questions that could be answered by appropriate research include:

1. What health care decisions do veterans and their families face, and what kinds of information needs do they have? How do they want to receive or access data about quality?
2. Are veterans aware of the VA's public reporting website? How often have they accessed the website? Do they understand the information being presented?
3. How well is VA's public reporting meeting Veteran needs?

Understanding this would help fashion transparency and public reporting efforts that provide the 'right' information at the 'right' time to the 'right' people. Key to achieving these goals may be the ability to tailor information to an individual, or to a subgroup of veterans. Health care decisions are personal, and generic information is unlikely to best provide what is wanted or needed. The combination of data, technology, and individualized information about potential health care service options and their implications presents the possibility of major improvements in public reporting.

REFERENCES

1. Open Government Plan, June 2010, Prepared on Behalf of the Honorable Eric K. Shinsheki, Secretary. United States Department of Veterans Affairs. 2010: Washington, D.C. p. 1-29.

2. VA Hospital Compare. November 23, 2010; Available from: http://www.hospitalcompare.va.gov/.

3. Berwick, D. M., B. James and M. J. Coye, Connections between quality measurement and improvement. Med Care, 2003. 41(1 Suppl): p. I30-8.

4. Hibbard, J. H., J. Stockard and M. Tusler, Hospital performance reports: impact on quality, market share, and reputation. Health Aff (Millwood), 2005. 24(4): p. 1150-60.

5. Fung, C. H., et al., Systematic review: the evidence that publishing patient care performance data improves quality of care. Ann Intern Med, 2008. 148(2): p. 111-23.

6. GRADE Working Group. Grading of Recommendations, Assessment, Development, and Evaluation. Available from: http://www.gradeworkinggroup.org/FAQ/index.htm.

7. Shea, B. J., et al., Development of AMSTAR: a measurement tool to assess the methodological quality of systematic reviews. BMC Med Res Methodol, 2007. 7: p. 10.

8. Marshall, M. N., et al., The public release of performance data - What do we expect to gain? A review of the evidence. Jama-Journal of the American Medical Association, 2000. 283(14): p. 1866-1874.

9. O'Neil, S., J. Schurrer and S. Simon, Environmental Scan of Public Reporting Programs and Analysis for the National Quality Forum. 2010, Mathematica Policy Research: Washington, D.C.

10. Hibbard, J. and S. Sofaer, Best practices in public reporting no. 1: how to effectively present health care performance data to consumers. June 2010, Agency for Healthcare Research and Quality: Rockville, MD. AHRQ Publication No. 10-0082-EF.

11. Sofaer, S. and J. Hibbard, Best practices in public reporting no. 2: Maximizing consumer understanding of public comparative quality reports: Effective use of explanatory information. June 2010, Agency for Healthcare Research and Quality: Rockville, MD. AHRQ Publication No. 10-0082-1-EF.

12. Sofaer, S. and J. Hibbard, Best practices in public reporting no. 3: How to maximize public awareness and use of comparative quality reports through effective promotion and dissemination strategies. June 2010, Agency for Healthcare Research and Quality: Rockville, MD. AHRQ Publication No. 10-0082-2-EF.

13. Overview: AHRQ Learning Network for Chartered Value Exchanges. September 2010; Available from: http://www.ahrq.gov/qual/value/lncveover.htm.

14.   Consumer Decision Points in Accessing Comparative Health Information. 2010, Robert
       Wood Johnson Foundation: Princeton, NJ.

15.   How to display comparative information that people can understand and use. 2010,
       Robert Wood Johnson Foundation: Princeton, NJ.

16.   About Aligning Forces for Quality. 2011; Available from: http://www.rwjf.org/
       qualityequality/af4q/about.jsp.

17.   Language to Use in Public Reporting About Hospital Care. 2011; Available from: http://
       www.rwjf.org/qualityequality/product.jsp?id=71839.

18.   How to Describe the Health and Community Context for Comparative Performance
       Reports 2011; Available from: http://www.rwjf.org/qualityequality/product.jsp?id=71842.

19.   Communicating with Physicians about Performance Measurement. 2011; Available from:
       http://www.rwjf.org/qualityequality/product.jsp?id=71803.

20.   Mazor, K. M., K. S. Dodd and L. Kunches, Communicating Hospital Infection Data
       to the Public: A Study of Consumer Responses and Preferences. American Journal of
       Medical Quality, 2009. 24(2): p. 108-115.

21.   Mazor, K. M. and K. S. Dodd, A Qualitative Study of Consumers' Views on Public
       Reporting of Health Care-Associated Infections. American Journal of Medical Quality,
       2009. 24(5): p. 412-418.

22.   Richard, S. A., S. Rawal and D. K. Martin, Patients' views about cardiac report cards: A
       qualitative study. Canadian Journal of Cardiology, 2005. 21(11): p. 943-947.

23.   Carman, K. L., Improving quality information in a consumer-driven era: showing the
       differences is crucial to informed consumer choice. Presentation at the 10th National
       CAHPS User Group Meeting. 2006: Baltimore, MD.

24.   Garcia-Lacalle, J., A bed too far - The implementation of freedom of choice policy in the
       NHS. Health Policy, 2008. 87(1): p. 31-40.

25.   Geraedts, M., D. Schwartze and T. Molzahn, Hospital quality reports in Germany: patient
       and physician opinion of the reported quality indicators. Bmc Health Services Research,
       2007. 7.

26.   Faber, M., et al., Public reporting in health care: how do consumers use quality-of-care
       information? A systematic review. Med Care, 2009. 47(1): p. 1-8.

27.   Dixon, A., J. Greene and J. Hibbard, Do consumer-directed health plans drive change in
       enrollees' health care behavior? Health Affairs, 2008. 27(4): p. 1120-1131.

28.   Peters, E., et al., Less is more in presenting quality information to consumers. Med Care
       Res Rev, 2007. 64: p. 169-190.

29.   Jha, A. K. and A. M. Epstein, The predictive accuracy of the New York State coronary
       artery bypass surgery report-card system. Health Aff (Millwood), 2006. 25(3): p. 844-55.

30.   Jin, G. Z. and A. T. Sorensen, Information and consumer choice: the value of publicized health plan ratings. J Health Econ, 2006. 25(2): p. 248-75.

31.   Uhrig, J. D., et al., Do content and format affect older consumers' use of comparative information in a Medicare health plan choice? Results from a controlled experiment. Med Care Res Rev, 2006. 63(6): p. 701-18.

32.   Cutler, D. A., R. S. Huckman and M. B. Landrum, The role of information in medical markets: An analysis of publicly reported outcomes in cardiac surgery. American Economic Review, 2004. 94(2): p. 342-346.

33.   Romano, P. S. and H. Zhou, Do well-publicized risk-adjusted outcomes reports affect hospital volume? Med Care, 2004. 42(4): p. 367-77.

34.   Baker, D. W., et al., The effect of publicly reporting hospital performance on market share and risk-adjusted mortality at high-mortality hospitals. Med Care, 2003. 41(6): p. 729-40.

35.   Beaulieu, N. D., Quality information and consumer health plan choices. J Health Econ, 2002. 21(1): p. 43-63.

36.   Chassin, M. R., Achieving and sustaining improved quality: lessons from New York State and cardiac surgery. Health Aff (Millwood), 2002. 21(4): p. 40-51.

37.   Farley, D. O., et al., Effects of CAHPS health plan performance information on plan choices by New Jersey Medicaid beneficiaries. Health Serv Res, 2002. 37(4): p. 985-1007.

38.   Farley, D. O., et al., Effect of CAHPS performance information on health plan choices by Iowa Medicaid beneficiaries. Med Care Res Rev, 2002. 59(3): p. 319-36.

39.   Harris, K. M., Can high quality overcome consumer resistance to restricted provider access? Evidence from a health plan choice experiment. Health Serv Res, 2002. 37(3): p. 551-71.

40.   Harris, K., J. Schultz and R. Feldman, Measuring consumer perceptions of quality differences among competing health benefit plans. Journal of Health Economics, 2002. 21(1): p. 1-17.

41.   Hibbard, J. H., et al., Strategies for reporting health plan performance information to consumers: evidence from controlled studies. Health Serv Res, 2002. 37(2): p. 291-313.

42.   Hibbard, J. H., et al., The impact of a CAHPS report on employee knowledge, beliefs, and decisions. Med Care Res Rev, 2002. 59(1): p. 104-16.

43.   Scanlon, D. P., et al., The impact of healthplan report cards on managed care enrollment. J Health Econ, 2002. 21: p. 19-41.

44.   Uhrig, J. D. and P. F. Short, Testing the effect of quality reports on the health plan choices of Medicare beneficiaries. Inquiry, 2002. 39(4): p. 355-71.

45.   Wedig, G. J. and M. Tai-Seale, The effect of report cards on consumer choice in the health insurance market. J Health Econ, 2002. 21(6): p. 1031-48.

46.   Hibbard, J. H., et al., Making health care quality reports easier to use. Jt Comm J Qual Improv, 2001. 27(11): p. 591-604.

47.   Schoenbaum, M., et al., Health plan choice and information about out-of-pocket costs: an experimental analysis. Inquiry, 2001. 38(1): p. 35-48.

48.   Hibbard, J. H., et al., Increasing the impact of health plan report cards by addressing consumers' concerns. Health Aff (Millwood), 2000. 19(5): p. 138-43.

49.   Spranca, M., et al., Do consumer reports of health plan quality affect health plan selection? Health Serv Res, 2000. 35(5 Pt 1): p. 933-47.

50.   Knutson, D. J., et al., Impact of report cards on employees: a natural experiment. Health Care Financ Rev, 1998. 20(1): p. 5-27.

51.   Mukamel, D. B. and A. I. Mushlin, Quality of care information makes a difference: an analysis of market share and price changes after publication of the New York State Cardiac Surgery Mortality Reports. Med Care, 1998. 36(7): p. 945-54.

52.   Mennemeyer, S. T., M. A. Morrisey and L. Z. Howard, Death and reputation: how consumers acted upon HCFA mortality information. Inquiry, 1997. 34(2): p. 117-28.

53.   Hibbard, J. H., S. Sofaer and J. J. Jewett, Condition-specific performance information: assessing salience, comprehension, and approaches for communicating quality. Health Care Financ Rev, 1996. 18(1): p. 95-109.

54.   Hannan, E. L., et al., New York State's Cardiac Surgery Reporting System: four years later. Ann Thorac Surg, 1994. 58(6): p. 1852-7.

55.   Vladeck, B. C., et al., Consumers and hospital use: the HCFA "death list". Health Aff (Millwood), 1988. 7(1): p. 122-5.

56.   Rainwater, J. A., et al., Evaluation of California's HMO report card: A report for the California Office of the Patient Advocate. 2005, UCD Center for Health Services Research in Primary Care: Davis, CA.

57.   Wang, J., et al., Do bad report cards have consequences? Impacts of publicly reported provider quality information on the CABG market in Pennsylvania. NBER Working Paper Series, 2010: p. 1-48.

58.   Hibbard, J. H., J. Stockard and M. Tusler, Does publicizing hospital performance stimulate quality improvement efforts? Health Aff (Millwood), 2003. 22(2): p. 84-94.

59.   Dziuban, S. W., Jr., et al., How a New York cardiac surgery program uses outcomes data. Ann Thorac Surg, 1994. 58(6): p. 1871-6.

60.   Bentley, J. M. and D. B. Nash, How Pennsylvania hospitals have responded to publicly released reports on coronary artery bypass graft surgery. Jt Comm J Qual Improv, 1998. 24(1): p. 40-9.

61.   Tu, J. V. and C. Cameron, Impact of an acute myocardial infarction report card in Ontario, Canada. Int J Qual Health Care, 2003. 15(2): p. 131-7.

62.   Rosenthal, G. E., et al., Using hospital performance data in quality improvement: the Cleveland Health Quality Choice experience. Jt Comm J Qual Improv, 1998. 24(7): p. 347-60.

63.   Longo, D. R., et al., Consumer reports in health care. Do they make a difference in patient care? JAMA, 1997. 278(19): p. 1579-84.

64.   Mannion, R., H. Davies and M. Marshall, Impact of star performance ratings in English acute hospital trusts. J Health Serv Res Policy, 2005. 10(1): p. 18-24.

65.   Luce, J. M., et al., Use of risk-adjusted outcome data for quality improvement by public hospitals. West J Med, 1996. 164(5): p. 410-4.

66.   Rainwater, J. A., P. S. Romano and D. M. Antonius, The California Hospital Outcomes Project: how useful is California's report card for quality improvement? Jt Comm J Qual Improv, 1998. 24(1): p. 31-9.

67.   Kim, C. Y., S. K. Ko and K. Y. Kim, Are league tables controlling epidemic of caesarean sections in South Korea? Bjog-an International Journal of Obstetrics and Gynaecology, 2005. 112(5): p. 607-611.

68.   Elliott, M. N., et al., Hospital Survey Shows Improvements In Patient Experience. Health Affairs, 2010. 29(11): p. 2061-2067.

69.   Hendriks, M., et al., Dutch healthcare reform: did it result in performance improvement of health plans? A comparison of consumer experiences over time. Bmc Health Services Research, 2009. 9.

70.   Bevan, G. and R. Hamblin, Hitting and missing targets by ambulance services for emergency calls: effects of different systems of performance measurement within the UK. Journal of the Royal Statistical Society Series a-Statistics in Society, 2009. 172: p. 161-190.

71.   Hannan, E. L., et al., Improving the outcomes of coronary artery bypass surgery in New York State. JAMA, 1994. 271(10): p. 761-6.

72.   Peterson, E. D., et al., The effects of New York's bypass surgery provider profiling on access to care and patient outcomes in the elderly. J Am Coll Cardiol, 1998. 32(4): p. 993-9.

73.   Ghali, W. A., et al., Statewide quality improvement initiatives and mortality after cardiac surgery. JAMA, 1997. 277(5): p. 379-82.

74.   Moscucci, M., et al., Public reporting and case selection for percutaneous coronary interventions: an analysis from two large multicenter percutaneous coronary intervention databases. J Am Coll Cardiol, 2005. 45(11): p. 1759-65.

75.   Omoigui, N. A., et al., Outmigration for coronary bypass surgery in an era of public dissemination of clinical outcomes. Circulation, 1996. 93(1): p. 27-33.

76.   Dranove, D., et al., Is more information better? The effects of "report cards" on health care providers. Journal of Political Economy, 2003. 111: p. 555-88.

77.   Rosenthal, G. E., L. Quinn and D. L. Harper, Declines in hospital mortality associated with a regional initiative to measure hospital performance. Am J Med Qual, 1997. 12(2): p. 103-12.

78.   Clough, J. D., et al., Lack of relationship between the Cleveland Health Quality Choice project and decreased inpatient mortality in Cleveland. Am J Med Qual, 2002. 17(2): p. 47-55.

79.   Baker, D. W., et al., Mortality trends during a program that publicly reported hospital performance. Med Care, 2002. 40(10): p. 879-90.

80.   Bost, J. E., Managed care organizations publicly reporting three years of HEDIS measures. Manag Care Interface, 2001. 14(9): p. 50-4.

81.   McCormick, D., et al., Relationship between low quality-of-care scores and HMOs' subsequent public disclosure of quality-of-care scores. JAMA, 2002. 288(12): p. 1484-90.

APPENDIX A. SEARCH STRATEGIES

The database was Web of Science; the sub-databases were Science (SCI-EXPANDED), Social Science (SSCI), Arts & Humanities (A&HCI) and the Science & Social Sciences Proceedings (CPCI-S & CPCI-SSH).

40 Cited Author=(epstein a*) AND Cited Year=(2000)
Databases=SCI-EXPANDED, SSCI, A&HCI, CPCI-S, CPCI-SSH Timespan=All Years

PMID- 10770153
TI - Public release of performance data: a progress report from the front.
AU - Epstein AM
PT - Comment
PT - Editorial
SO - JAMA. 2000 Apr 12;283(14):1884-6.

268 Cited Author=(epstein a*) AND Cited Year=(1998)
Databases=SCI-EXPANDED, SSCI, A&HCI, CPCI-S, CPCI-SSH Timespan=All Years

PMID- 9624015
TI - Rolling down the runway: the challenges ahead for quality report cards.
AU - Epstein AM
SO - JAMA. 1998 Jun 3;279(21):1691-6.

197 Cited Author=(schneider e*) AND Cited Year=(1996)
Databases=SCI-EXPANDED, SSCI, A&HCI, CPCI-S, CPCI-SSH Timespan=All Years

PMID- 8657242
TI - Influence of cardiac-surgery performance reports on referral practices and access to care. A survey of cardiovascular specialists.
AU - Schneider EC
AU - Epstein AM
SO - N Engl J Med. 1996 Jul 25;335(4):251-6.

180 Cited Author=(schneider e*) AND Cited Year=(1998)
Databases=SCI-EXPANDED, SSCI, A&HCI, CPCI-S, CPCI-SSH Timespan=All Years

PMID- 9613914
TI - Use of public performance reports: a survey of patients undergoing cardiac surgery.
AU - Schneider EC
AU - Epstein AM
SO - JAMA. 1998 May 27;279(20):1638-42.

104 Cited Author=(fung c*) AND Cited Year=(2008)
Databases=SCI-EXPANDED, SSCI, A&HCI, CPCI-S, CPCI-SSH Timespan=All Years

Fung, C. H., Y. W. Lim, S. Mattke, C. Damberg and P. G. Shekelle. "Systematic review: the evidence that publishing patient care performance data improves quality of care." Ann Intern Med 148(2): 111-23.

412 Cited Author=(marshall m*) AND Cited Year=(2000)
Databases=SCI-EXPANDED, SSCI, A&HCI, CPCI-S, CPCI-SSH Timespan=All Years

2000. Marshall, M. N., P. G. Shekelle, R. H. Brook and S. Leatherman. "Use of performance data to change physician behavior." JAMA 284(9): 1079.

2000. Marshall, M. N., P. G. Shekelle, S. Leatherman and R. H. Brook. "The public release of performance data: what do we expect to gain? A review of the evidence." JAMA 283(14): 1866-74.

2000. Marshall, M. N., P. G. Shekelle, S. Leatherman and R. H. Brook. "Public disclosure of performance data: learning from the US experience." Quality in Health Care 9(1): 53-57.

2000. Dying to Know: Public Release of Information about Quality of Health Care by Martin Marshall, Paul G. Shekelle, Robert H. Brook, Sheila Leatherman. RAND MR-1255

APPENDIX B. STUDY SELECTION FORM

1. **Included in Fung or 2006 and earlier**
   Included in Fung .... STOP
   2006 or earlier .... ☐

2. **What types of health care setting are the quality and safety information about?**
   Health plan/ HMO .... ☐
   Health system .... ☐
   Hospital .... ☐
   Physician/ Individual providers .... STOP
   Other, specify: .... _____

3. **Which Key Question* does this article address?**
   KQ1 .... ☐
   KQ2 .... ☐
   KQ3 .... ☐
   KQ4 .... ☐
   None .... STOP
   Background .... STOP

   > * KQ1: What is known about the most effective way of displaying quality and safety information, comparative
   > data about health system structure, services, and performance so that it is understandable?
   > KQ2: How do patients prefer to receive or access this information?
   > KQ3: What is the evidence that patients or their families use publicly reported quality and safety information
   > to make informed health care decisions?
   > KQ4: What is the evidence that public reporting of quality and safety information leads to improved quality
   > or safety?

4. **What is the study design?**
   RCT .... ☐
   Observational, concurrent comparison .... ☐
   Observational, time series (no concurrent) .... ☐
   Observational, other .... ☐
   Systematic Review .... ☐
   Non-systematic review, commentary or news, other .... STOP
   Misc include .... _____

5. **Does this article discuss one of the following report cards/ reported data?**
   New York State Reporting System .... ☐
   CAHPS .... ☐
   HEDIS .... ☐
   Cleveland .... ☐
   Wisconsin .... ☐
   Medicare compare .... ☐
   California .... ☐
   Other, specify: .... _____

6. **What country is the data from?**
   US .... ☐
   Europe .... ☐
   Canada .... ☐
   Australia/New Zealand .... ☐
   Other, specify: ...._____
   Unclear/not stated .... ☐

7. **What level do the data come from?**
   National or sufficiently representative .... ☐
   Regional .... ☐
   Single state .... ☐
   City/county .... ☐
   Single medical center .... ☐
   Unknown .... ☐

What outcomes are reported?

8. **Individual-level outcomes**
   Health/clinic outcomes .... ☐
   Patient selection of plan or provider .... ☐
   Patient satisfaction .... ☐
   Provider satisfaction .... ☐
   Patient-provider communication .... ☐
   Self-management .... ☐
   Adherence (medication, visit) .... ☐
   Provider practice patterns .... ☐
   Harms or benefits .... ☐
   Other, specify: ...._____

9. **System-level outcomes**
   Quality improvement activity .... ☐
   Change in quality rating/scores .... ☐
   Efficiency .... ☐
   Privacy breaches .... ☐
   Patient safety .... ☐
   Attitudes .... ☐
   Usability .... ☐
   Harms or benefits .... ☐
   Other, specify: ...._____

APPENDIX C. EVIDENCE TABLES FOR KEY QUESTIONS #1 AND #2

Author, Year (ID)	Objective	Subject of public reporting; Hospital/ Health plan; Location	Sample	Design Type	Design Rating; Global Rating	Key Findings
Mazor, 2009[20]	To evaluate consumers' responses to different approaches to public reporting of comparative hospital data on HAIs.	Healthcare-associated Infections (HAIs); Hospital; Worcester, MA	Random sample of residents; 201 completed surveys; Response rate 34% of those sent to valid addresses; 25% of all selected addresses. Age: Mean 51.7; 37.8% male; 28.4% HS education or less	Experiment (random sample; random assignment of versions of mock report)	4;2	The three report characteristics tested (consistency of hospital rating across indicators included; presenting results in words or charts, and including confidence intervals) had no significant impact on understandability. More respondents with a higher level of education (at least some college) rated 2 sections of the report as easier to understand verse those with high school education or less. For the other 5 sections the differences between education levels were not statistically significant. Age was not found to effect understandability.
Mazor, 2009[21]	To understand consumer response to public reports and how reports might be improved.	HAIs; Hospital; Worcester, MA	Random sample of residents; 59 participants; 22 (37.3%) male; age range 24-82; mean 53.3; 25.4% high school education or less	In-depth interviews; random sample of residents invited to participant.	2;2	Most respondents had no prior knowledge/understanding of HCI and this required explanation before different reports could be discussed. Inconsistent rankings across hospitals made it difficult for interviewees to pick the 'best' hospital. Format: number preferred over symbols; confidence intervals were confusing; interviewees unable to paraphrase definition of risk adjustment provided in the mock reports; print preferred to internet.
Richard, 2005[22]	To use qualitative interviews to understand patients' views of report cards on cardiac care.	Cardiac report cards; Hospital; Canada	7 cities with major cardiac programs; 91 cardiac patients	63 individual interviews and 6 focus groups	2;2	Participants endorsed the idea of report cards, wanted to see improvement in report card scores over time, and would use them if relevant. Patients wanted report cards to contain additional information to supplement the traditional outcomes (e.g., mortality, morbidity), specifically the experiences of other cardiac patients and non-medical aspects of care. Dissemination ideas were varied and included important roles for family physicians and cardiologist to provide and explain the report cards.

Design ratings: 4 stars indicate a strong study design rating; while 1 star indicates a weaker study design rating.
Global ratings: 3 indicates great weight in the stratum's body of evidence; and 1 indicates little weight.

APPENDIX D. EVIDENCE TABLES FOR KEY QUESTION #3

Author, Year (ID)	Objective	Subject of public reporting; Hospital/Health plan; Location	Sample	Design Type	Design Rating; Global Rating	Key Findings
Articles from Fung and colleagues						
Farley, 2002[37]	To assess effects of providing CAHPS information on plan choices	CAHPS; Health plan; New Jersey	HMO Medical Plans in New Jersey; Medicaid beneficiaries (1998)	Randomized controlled trial	4;3	No effect on HMO choices overall; Participants who read the report card and did not select the dominant HMO chose the HMO with higher CAHPS scores.
Farley, 2002[38]	To assess effects of providing CAHPS information on plan choices	CAHPS; Health plan; Iowa	HMO Medical Plans in Iowa; Medicaid Beneficiaries (2000)	Randomized controlled trial	4;2	No effect on HMO choices overall
Spranca, 2000[49]	To assess effects of providing CAHPS information about hypothetical health plans on plan choices	Hypothetical plans; Health plan; Los Angeles	Hypothetical plans in laboratory setting; adults with private insurance	Experimental study	4;2	When plans had high CAHPS ratings, participants were willing to enroll in less expensive plans that restrict services
Harris, 2002[39]	To investigate the impact of expert-assessed and consumer-assessed quality ratings on willingness to enroll in hypothetical health plans that restrict provider access	Hypothetical plans; Health plan; Los Angeles	Laboratory setting; Privately insured adults (2000)	Experimental study	4;2	Provision of report cards with information about quality of health plan reduced importance of provider network features
Beaulieu, 2002[35]	To assess effects of providing health plan performance data (HEDIS measures, patient satisfaction) on consumers' enrollment decisions	HEDIS; Health plan; Harvard University	Private health plans available to Harvard employees; Harvard employees (1994 to 1997)	Observational cohort	3;2	Provision of quality information had a small but statistically significant effect on health plan choices.
Wedig, 2002[45]	To assess effects of providing quality ratings from the Federal Employee Health Benefit guide on consumers' plan choices	Federal Employee Health Benefit guide; Health plan; U.S.	Private health plans available to federal employees; Federal employees with single person HMO coverage residing in counties with 5 or fewer unique plans (1995 to 1996)	Observational cohort	3;2	Dissemination of report cards influenced plan selection. Employees were more likely to select plans with better quality ratings.

Design ratings: 4 stars indicate a strong study design rating; while 1 star indicates a weaker study design rating.
Global ratings: 3 indicates great weight in the stratum's body of evidence; and 1 indicates little weight.

Public Presentation of Health System or Facility Data about Quality and Safety: A Systematic Review

Author, Year (ID)	Objective	Subject of public reporting; Hospital/Health plan; Location	Sample	Design Type	Design Rating; Global Rating	Key Findings
Jin, 2005[30]	To assess effects of providing quality ratings from the Federal Employee Health Benefit guide on plan choices	Federal Employee Health Benefit guide; Health plan; U.S.	Private health plans serving federal employees; Federal employees, retirees, and surviving family of deceased federal employees (1998-1999)	Observational cohort	3;3	Overall, inertia in health plan enrollment decisions. For individuals affected by performance ratings, better scores were associated with increased likelihood of selecting the plan.
Scanlon, 2002[43]	To assess effects of providing HEDIS and patient satisfaction ratings on plan choices	HEDIS; Health plan; General Motors;	General Motors employees (1996-1997); Private health plans (HMO only)	Observational cohort	3;3	Employees avoided plans with many below average ratings and would be willing to pay more to avoid plans with lower ratings, but were not strongly attracted to plans with many superior ratings.
Mennemeyer, 1997[52]	To assess the relationship between the release of HCFA hospital-specific mortality rates and utilization (discharges); to compare the impact of releasing HCFA mortality rates to press reports of unexpected deaths, on utilizations.	HCFA; Hospital; U.S.	Community hospitals treating Medicare patients (1984-1992)	Observational cohort	3;2	Hospitals with mortality rates two times that expected by HCFA had less than one fewer discharge per week in the first year; press reports of single, unexpected deaths was associated with 9% reduction in hospital discharges within one year.
Vladeck, 1988[55]	To examine relationship between mortality rate outlier status and hospital CABG volume/quality improvement activity following CSRS implementation	NYS CSRS; Hospital; New York	All New York general acute hospitals serving Medicare patients (~1985 to ~1986)	Analysis of Time Trend	2;1	No significant effect on occupancy rates
Mukamel, 1998[51]	To measure the relationship between provider (hospital, physician) ratings in the CSRS and rates of growth in fee-for-service market share	NYS CSRS; Hospital; New York	All New York hospitals performing CABG (1990 to 1993)	Observational cohort	2;1	Hospitals with better outcomes experienced higher rates of growth in market share
Hannan, 1994[54]	To determine if mortality rate outlier status was associated with overall improvement in risk-adjusted mortality and changes in provider volume of CABG operations performed following the implementation of the CSRS	NYS CSRS; Hospital; New York	All New York hospital performing CABG (1989 to 1992)	Observational cohort	3;2	No association between mortality rate outlier status and hospital volume

Design ratings: 4 stars indicate a strong study design rating; while 1 star indicates a weaker study design rating.
Global ratings: 3 indicates great weight in the stratum's body of evidence; and 1 indicates little weight.

Author, Year (ID)	Objective	Subject of public reporting; Hospital/Health plan; Location	Sample	Design Type	Design Rating; Global Rating	Key Findings
Chassin, 2002[36]	To examine relationship between mortality rate outlier status and hospital CABG volume/quality improvement activity following the CSRS implementation	NYS CSRS; Hospital; New York	New York hospitals with the highest and lowest CABG mortality from 1989-1995	Analysis of Time Trend	2;1	Small changes in market share and less than half the time in the expected direction
Jha, 2006[29]	To examine the relationship between providers' CSRS rankings and market share; to examine impact of cardiac surgeons' performance on the likelihood of ceasing practice in New York	NYS CSRS; Hospital; New York	All New York hospitals performing CABG for more than 3 years (1989 to 2002)	Time Series (for market share analysis)	3;2	No significant relationship between ranking and subsequent market share
Baker, 2003[34]	To examine market share following the release of risk-adjusted 30-day mortality rates for six acute conditions as part of the CHQC program	CHQC; Hospital; Northeast Ohio	30 nonfederal hospitals (1991 to 1997)	Time Series	3;2	No statistically significant relationship overall between higher than expected mortality rates and market share
Romano, 2004[33]	To examine the relationship between outlier status in California & New York public reports in three conditions/ procedures (CABG mortality in New York, AMI and postdiskectomy complications in California) and hospital volume	NYS CSRS and CA; New York and California	All licensed hospitals in New York State performing CABG, non-federal hospitals in California except Kaiser hospitals and state developmental and correctional hospitals	Time Series	3;2	No significant AMI-related volume changes among outlier hospitals. Slight increase in lumbar diskectomy-related volume for low-complication outliers. Significant transient increase in CABG volume for low-mortality hospitals and transient decrease in volume for high-mortality outliers.
Hibbard, 2005[4]	To compare the impact of public (QualityCounts), internal (private) and no reporting on quality improvement activity, market share, and risk-adjusted performance (three clinical areas--hip/knee surgery, cardiac care, and obstetric care)	QualityCounts; Hospital; South central Wisconsin	Hospitals participating in Quality Counts; 24 Hospitals	Analysis of Time Trend	2;2	No significant changes in market share for hospital with publicly-reported data. No results given for internal or no reporting groups.

Design ratings: 4 stars indicate a strong study design rating; while 1 star indicates a weaker study design rating.
Global ratings: 3 indicates great weight in the stratum's body of evidence; and 1 indicates little weight.

Author, Year (ID)	Objective	Subject of public reporting; Hospital/Health plan; Location	Sample	Design Type	Design Rating; Global Rating	Key Findings
New articles not in Fung and colleagues						
Cutler, 2004[32]	To examine whether where patients go for bypass surgery (the distribution of patients across providers) affected by report cards	NYS CSRS; Hospital, New York State	All hospitals performing bypass surgery in New York (3,406 patients in the baseline year)	Observational, time series– across hospital rather than statewide trends.	3;3	Hospitals identified as high-mortality by the report experienced an approximated 10% decline in bypass surgery (4.9 fewer patients with hospital averages of 50 surgeries per month, significant at the 0.5 level); while low mortality hospitals do not experience an increase. The reduction is in low-severity, not high severity patients.
Harris, 2002[40]	To determine if consumers perceive the quality of health plans and how quality relates to their choice of health plan.	N/A; Health plan; Minneapolis and St. Paul, MN	Randomly-selected eligible employees interviewed by phone. 721 interviewed. 91% response rate. Limited to unmarried employees with no dependents	Observational: cross sectional	3;2	Incorporating information from consumers about how important to them different attributes of health plans are improves models that explain health plan choice.
Dixon, 2008[27]	To examine the influence of health plan (consumer driven health plan versus preferred provider organization) on the use of health-related information and health services	N/A; Health plan; Large manufacturing company	Health plan/HMO; US; Employees of a large manufacturing company	Observational, time series (no concurrent)	2;1	Enrollees in lower-deductible CDHP were most likely to start using information. Enrollees in high-deductible CDHP were more likely to use cost information than PPO enrollees. Variation in information seeking decreased throughout study.

Design ratings: 4 stars indicate a strong study design rating; while 1 star indicates a weaker study design rating.
Global ratings: 3 indicates great weight in the stratum's body of evidence; and 1 indicates little weight.

APPENDIX E. EVIDENCE TABLES FOR KEY QUESTION #4

Author, Year (ID)	Objective	Subject of public reporting; Hospital/Health plan; Location	Sample	Design Type	Design Rating; Global Rating	Key Findings
Impact on Quality Improvement Activity Articles from Fung						
Chassin, 2002[36]	To examine relationship between mortality rate outlier status and hospital CABG volume/quality improvement activity following the implementation of the CSRS	NYS CSRS; Hospital; New York State	Key informants at four hospitals and state officials directly involved in efforts to quality improvement efforts at the hospitals	Case Series	1;1	Increase in quality improvement activity (e.g., staffing policy changes, multidisciplinary approach to examining care processes, changes in operating room schedule)
Dziuban, 1994[59]	To document a hospital's response to being identified as a high risk-adjusted mortality outlier in the CSRS	NYS CSRS; Hospital; New York State	One outlier hospital	Case Study	1;1	Quality improvement activity increased (change in timing & technique used for patients undergoing emergent CABG, change in hospital policies)
Bentley, 1998[60]	To determine whether Pennsylvania Health Care Cost Containment Council's Consumer Guide to CABG, which compared in-hospital mortality rates, led to more changes in Pennsylvania hospitals' CABG policies/practices than in New Jersey hospitals, which were not required to publicly-report performance results	Pennsylvania consumer guide; Hospital; Pennsylvania and New Jersey	Key informants at the hospitals identified by the chief executive officers of these hospitals; Hospitals providing CABG surgery	Survey (Descriptive)	1;1	Response in Pennsylvania hospitals (e.g., recruited staff, started continuous quality improvement program to improve CABG procedures). More changes in Pennsylvania than New Jersey hospitals (no formal statistical testing because small sample size)
Hibbard, 2003[58]	To compare the effects of public reporting (QualityCounts) to confidential reporting and no reporting, on quality improvement activity, market share (hospital discharges), and risk-adjusted performance (two summary indices of adverse events and indices in three clinical areas--hip/knee surgery, cardiac care, and obstetric care)	QualityCounts; Hospital; South central Wisconsin	Hospitals participating in Quality Counts (n=24)	Controlled Before/After Trial	3;1	Compared to hospitals that received confidential reports or no reports, QualityCounts hospital did not engage in more quality improvements overall, but they did engage in a statistically higher number of quality improvement efforts specific to the areas included in the reports.

Design ratings: 4 stars indicate a strong study design rating; while 1 star indicates a weaker study design rating.
Global ratings: 3 indicates great weight in the stratum's body of evidence; and 1 indicates little weight.

Public Presentation of Health System or Facility Data about Quality and Safety: A Systematic Review

Evidence-based Synthesis Program

Author, Year (ID)	Objective	Subject of public reporting; Hospital/Health plan; Location	Sample	Design Type	Design Rating; Global Rating	Key Findings
Hibbard, 2005[4]	To compare the impact of public (QualityCounts), internal (private) and no reporting, on quality improvement activity, market share (hospital discharges), and risk-adjusted performance (two summary indices of adverse events and indices in three clinical areas--hip/knee surgery, cardiac care, and obstetric care)	QualityCounts; Hospital; South central Wisconsin	Hospitals participating in Quality Counts (n=24)	Descriptive (survey) (for quality improvement analysis)	1;1	Out of seven possible activities, mean number of quality improvement activities was 4.1 overall; 5.7 for hospitals with improved ratings; 2.6 with no change in ratings; 4 with decrease in ratings (no formal statistical testing)
Rosenthal, 1998[62]	To study quality improvement activities following release of CHQC reports of mortality rates, length of stay, and cesarean section rates (all measures severity-adjusted)	CHQC; Hospital; Cleveland	One academic and three community hospitals of varying size in the Cleveland area	Case Series	1;1	Quality improvement activities increased (e.g., interdisciplinary process improvement teams, detailed review of processes of care, development of practice guidelines)
Tu, 2003[61]	To study the impact of the "Cardiovascular Health and Services in Ontario: AN ICES Atlas," which reports hospital-specific acute myocardial infarction performance measures, on quality improvement activity	ICES; Hospital; Ontario, Canada	All Ontario hospitals providing acute myocardial infarction care; Physicians working in Ontario hospitals representing 62 of 121 eligible hospitals (52% overall hospital response rate)	Descriptive (survey)	1;1	54% of respondents indicated that one or more changes were made at their hospital
Longo, 1997[63]	To examine the impact of Missouri Department of Health's obstetrics consumer report, which provides structure, process, and outcomes measures, on quality improvement activity and clinical outcomes	MO Dept. Health obstetrics consumer report; Hospital; Missouri	All hospitals providing obstetric care; Key informant designated by hospital administrators at 82 hospitals (93% response rate)	Descriptive (survey)	1;1	Hospitals instituted services (e.g., hospital policy for that infants ride in car seats upon discharge, formal neonatal transfer agreements) after the reports were published
Luce, 1996[65]	To describe quality improvement activity following the California OSHPD's CHOP report featuring risk-adjusted outcomes	OSHPD CHOP; Hospital; California	All California non-federal hospitals; 17 out of 22 public hospitals that are members of the California Association of Public Hospitals and Health Systems	Descriptive (survey)	1;1	Minimal impact on quality improvement activity

Design ratings: 4 stars indicate a strong study design rating; while 1 star indicates a weaker study design rating.
Global ratings: 3 indicates great weight in the stratum's body of evidence; and 1 indicates little weight.

44

Author, Year (ID)	Objective	Subject of public reporting; Hospital/Health plan; Location	Sample	Design Type	Design Rating; Global Rating	Key Findings
Rainwater, 1998[66]	To describe the impact of publicly reporting California's CHOP risk-adjusted 30-day inpatient mortality rates for patients with acute myocardial infarction, on quality improvement activity	OSHPD CHOP; Hospital; California	California non-federal acute care hospitals; 39 key informants at a sample of acute care hospitals in California	Interviews	1;1	Minimal impact on quality improvement activity (2/3 respondents indicated no specific QI activity)
Mannion, 2005[64]	To describe impact of the National Health Service (NHS) star performance ratings on quality improvement efforts	NHS; Hospital; United Kingdom	All hospital trusts; Staff at four low performing hospital trusts and two high performing hospital trusts	Case series	1;1	Ratings transmitted important priorities from central government and helped direct and concentrate front-line resources. Public reporting led to tunnel vision and distortion of clinical priorities and disincentive to improve performance among high-rated organizations.
Impact on Quality Improvement Articles, not in Fung						
Wang, 2010[57]	To examine the impact of report cards on provider volume (hospital and surgeons) and on patient matching with surgeons.	Hospital CABG Volume	Hospitals in PA who perform 30 or more CABG per year between 3rd Q 1998 and 1st Q 2006	Observational Cohort	3; 2	Report cards have no significant impact on hospital surgical volume and do not change the population of patients who have CABG. Report cards have a larger impact on the distribution of healthier patients as opposed to sicker across hospitals. Bad rating takes a year to have an effect on volume which was estimated as a decrease in quarterly CABG cases of about 15%. These were almost all among low severity CABG cases. This effect did not persist past one year.

Design ratings: 4 stars indicate a strong study design rating; while 1 star indicates a weaker study design rating.
Global ratings: 3 indicates great weight in the stratum's body of evidence; and 1 indicates little weight.

Author, Year (ID)	Objective	Subject of public reporting; Hospital/Health plan; Location	Sample	Design Type	Design Rating; Global Rating	Key Findings
Rainwater, 2005[56]	To evaluate the use and impact of California's Quality of Care Report Card (QRC), based on three questions: 1. Do consumers use the QRC? 2. How useful to consumers are the quality measures included in the QRC? 3. What is the impact of the QRC on quality improvement and other activities in the participating HMOs and medical groups?	California's Quality of Care Report Card (QRC); Health Plan; California	6 consumer focus groups, 2,341 respondents to mail and internet surveys, 56 key informants	Mixed methods: focus groups, surveys, interviews	3;3	Use is reported at over 28,000 visitors to the QRC website annually, and over 100,000 booklets distributed. Users are most interested in comparing HMOs in the plan service domain, and find features like the specialty care information, specific measures such as mental health care, and comparative performance information by health topic or disease most helpful.
Impact on Clinical Outcomes Articles From Fung						
Hannan, 1994[71]	To assess changes in in-hospital mortality rates of CABG patients following the publication of mortality data in the CSRS	NYS CSRS; Hospital; New York	All New York hospitals performing CABG; 57187 patients undergoing CABG (1989-1992)	Analysis of Time Trend	2;2	RAMR decreased from 4.17% to 2.45%.
Dziuban, 1994[59]	To document a hospital's response to being identified as a high risk-adjusted mortality outlier in the CSRS	NYS CSRS; Hospital; New York	One poor performing hospital	Case Study	1;1	Excess mortality was localized to high-acuity patients undergoing emergent CABG. Mortality decreased to zero following focused effort to optimize management of these patients.
Hannan, 1994[54]	To determine if mortality rate outlier status was associated with changes in CABG-related in-hospital risk-adjusted mortality rates following the implementation of the CSRS	NYS CSRS; Hospital; New York	All New York hospitals performing CABG; All New York patients discharged after CABG (1989 to 1992)	Analysis of Time Trend	2;2	Reductions in RAMR, especially among hospitals that had highest initial mortality rates. Convergence in risk-adjusted mortality rates among hospitals initially identified as high, medium, and low performers.
Peterson, 1998[72]	To examine the impact of the CSRS on in-hospital mortality rates by comparing unadjusted mortality rates in New York to other states. To examine the impact of the CSRS on in-state access to CABG and referral out-of-state of patients in need of CABG	NYS CSRS; Hospital; New York	All hospitals performing CABG; Medicare patients 65 or older who underwent CABG in a U.S. hospital (1987 to 1992)	Observational cohort	3;3	Both unadjusted and risk-adjusted mortality rates in New York declined more than in other states. NY MI patients were less likely to receive CABG, but the overall percentage of NY MI patients receiving CABG rose, paralleling national trends, even among higher risk elderly subsets; out-of-state CABG rates declined

Design ratings: 4 stars indicate a strong study design rating; while 1 star indicates a weaker study design rating.
Global ratings: 3 indicates great weight in the stratum's body of evidence; and 1 indicates little weight.

Public Presentation of Health System or Facility Data about Quality and Safety: A Systematic Review

Author, Year (ID)	Objective	Subject of public reporting; Hospital/Health plan; Location	Sample	Design Type	Design Rating; Global Rating	Key Findings
Ghali, 1997[73]	To compare trends in CABG-related mortality in Massachusetts (a state without statewide public reporting of CABG outcomes) to New York (a state with public reporting) and northern New England	NYS CSRS; Hospitals; New York and Massachusetts	All NY hospitals performing CABG; 12 Massachusetts hospitals performing cardiac surgery (except Veterans Affairs hospitals) and hospitals contained in the HCFA hospital 30-day unadjusted mortality dataset (1990, 1992, and 1994)	Observational cohort	3;2	RAMR reductions in Massachusetts were comparable to mortality reduction in New York and northern New England; unadjusted mortality trends were similar in Massachusetts, New York, northern New England, and the United States
Rosenthal, 1997[77]	To measure changes in hospital mortality that occurred following the implementation of the CHQC reporting initiative, which publicly-released in-hospital mortality rates	CHQC; Hospital; Cleveland	Hospitals in the Cleveland area; 101,060 consecutive eligible discharges with eight diagnoses (acute myocardial infarction, heart failure, obstructive airway disease, gastrointestinal hemorrhage, pneumonia, stroke, CABG, and lower bowel resection) from 30 northeastern Ohio hospitals (1992 to 1993)	Time Series	3;1	Risk-adjusted mortality for most conditions declined from 7.5% to 6.8%, 6.8%, and 6.5% for 3 periods following publication. Declines in mortality rates were significant in weighted linear regression analyses for heart failure (0.50% per period) and pneumonia (0.38% per period)
Baker, 2003[34]	To examine hospitals' market share and 30-day risk-adjusted mortality at hospitals participating in CHQC	CHQC; Hospital; Cleveland	Medicare patients receiving care at these Cleveland-area hospitals (1991 to 1997)	Time Series	3;2	Hospital outlier status was not significantly related to changes in risk-adjusted 30-day mortality between 1991 and 1997.
Clough, 2002[78]	To measure changes in in-hospital mortality rates associated with the implementation of the CHQC reporting initiative	CHQC; Hospital; Cleveland	Hospitals included in the Ohio Hospital Association's inpatient discharge data (1992 to 1995)	Observational cohort	3;2	No statistical difference in rate of decline in combined mortality in Cleveland compared to the rest of the Ohio
Longo, 1997[63]	To examine the impact of Missouri Department of Health's obstetrics consumer report, which provides structure, process, and outcomes measures	MO Dept. Health obstetrics consumer report; Hospital; Missouri	All Missouri hospitals providing obstetrics care (1989 to 1993)	Observational cohort	3;2	Improvements in ultrasound rates, vaginal birth after cesarean rates, and cesarean rates were noted among outlier hospitals

Design ratings: 4 stars indicate a strong study design rating; while 1 star indicates a weaker study design rating.
Global ratings: 3 indicates great weight in the stratum's body of evidence; and 1 indicates little weight.

Author, Year (ID)	Objective	Subject of public reporting; Hospital/Health plan; Location	Sample	Design Type	Design Rating; Global Rating	Key Findings
Hibbard, 2005[4]	To compare the impact of public (QualityCounts), internal (private) and no reporting, on quality improvement activity, market share (hospital discharges), and risk-adjusted performance (two summary indices of adverse events and indices in three clinical areas--hip/knee surgery, cardiac care, and obstetric care)	QualityCounts; Hospital; South central Wisconsin	Hospitals participating in Quality Counts (2001 to 2003, n=24)	Controlled Before/After Trial (for outcomes analysis)	3;2	Performance feedback, whether public or private, was associated with improved performance
Moscucci, 2005[74]	To measure the effect of the New York State PCI report on case selection for percutaneous coronary intervention (PCI) by comparing Michigan's and New York's adjusted and unadjusted in-hospital mortality rates	NYS PCI (CSRS); Hospital; New York and Michigan	All New York hospitals performing CABG; 11,374 patients in a multicenter (eight hospital) PCI database in Michigan and 69,048 patients in a statewide (34 hospital) PCI database in New York (1998 to 1999)	Observational cohort	3;2	Unadjusted mortality rates were significantly lower in New York than Michigan, but adjusted mortality rates were not statistically different.
Omoigui, 1996[75]	To determine if dissemination of CSRS mortality data was associated with outmigration of high-risk patients to undergo treatment at the Cleveland Clinic	NYS CSRS; Hospital; New York and Cleveland	All hospital performing CABG in New York State; 9,442 patients receiving CABG at the Cleveland Clinic (1989 to 1993)	Observational cohort	3;2	Patients from New York State receiving CABG at the Cleveland Clinic had higher RAMR than patients from Ohio, other states, and other countries
Dranove, 2003[76]	To study the effects of public reporting in New York and Pennsylvania	NYS CSRS and Pennsylvania public reporting system; Hospital; New York and Pennsylvania	All New York and Pennsylvania hospitals performing CABG; Medicare beneficiaries and hospitals found in a Medicare claims data set (not specified) and hospitals participating in the American Hospital Association annual survey (1987 to 1994)	Observational cohort	3;2	Report cards shifted CABG use to healthier patients, leading to worse outcomes, especially among sicker patients (defined as higher hospital expenditures and days in hospital)

Design ratings: 4 stars indicate a strong study design rating; while 1 star indicates a weaker study design rating.
Global ratings: 3 indicates great weight in the stratum's body of evidence; and 1 indicates little weight.

Author, Year (ID)	Objective	Subject of public reporting; Hospital/Health plan; Location	Sample	Design Type	Design Rating; Global Rating	Key Findings
Baker, 2002[79]	To examine mortality trends associated with the CHQC program	CHQC; Hospital; Cleveland	Hospitals in the Cleveland area; Medicare patients hospitalized with acute myocardial infarction, heart failure, gastrointestinal hemorrhage, obstructive pulmonary disease, pneumonia, or stroke (1991 to 1999)	Time Series	3;2	Risk-adjusted in-hospital mortality declined significantly for most conditions, but the mortality rate in the early post discharge period rose significantly for most conditions and the 30-day mortality rate declined significantly for only heart failure and obstructive pulmonary disease
Bost, 2001[80]	To compare HEDIS and CAHPS results for plans that publicly report data with those who do not, over a three-year period	HEDIS and CAHPS; Health plan U.S.	Commercial health plans (1997-1999)	Observational cohort	2;1	Technical performance measures and patient experience measures (except communication) were higher for health plans that publicly report data.
McCormick, 2002[81]	To assess the relationship between health plan performance and participation in public reporting programs	HMO commercial health plans; Health plan; U.S.	HMO health plans (1997 to 1999)	Observational cohort	2;2	Lower-scoring plans are significantly more likely than plans with higher-scoring plans to stop disclosing publicly their quality data
Impact on Clinical Outcomes Articles, not in Fung						
Bevan, 2009[70]	To assess the impact of public reporting on the performance of ambulance services	Ambulance service response times; UK	Yearly data from 2000 to 2005	"natural experiment" Comparison of UK countries with the same target but one had reporting and the others did not.	3;2	Response times improved in the countries with public reporting and did not in others. Examination of potential harms found evidence that some types of gaming occurred (data was changed) but that others types that were suspected (changes in the classification of the event) did not.
Cutler, 2004[32]	To examine whether medical quality among hospitals are affected by report cards	NYS CSRS; Hospital; New York State	All hospitals performing bypass surgery in New York (3,406 patients in the baseline year)	Observational, time series–across hospital rather than statewide trends.	3;2	Hospitals identified as high mortality improve performance in terms of decreased risk-adjusted mortality rates: mortality declined 1.2 percentage points (significant at the 0.01 level) in these low quality hospitals during the 12 months after the reporting.

Design ratings: 4 stars indicate a strong study design rating; while 1 star indicates a weaker study design rating.
Global ratings: 3 indicates great weight in the stratum's body of evidence; and 1 indicates little weight.

Author, Year (ID)	Objective	Subject of public reporting; Hospital/Health plan; Location	Sample	Design Type	Design Rating; Global Rating	Key Findings
Elliott, 2010[68]	To determine if hospitals improved in terms of patient experience over the initial 2 years of public reporting of HCAHPS results	HCAHPS; Hospital; US	Hospital, National CAHPS US 61% of hospitals in 3/08 3,864; 84 % of hospitals in 3/09 3,863 Patient response rate averaged 34%--patients are a random sample of discharges	Observational, Time series, no comparison group	3;2	Hospitals improved in 8 of 9 domains as measured by percent of positive responses (MD communication did not improve). Magnitude of changes was small, but would result in change in ranking. Hospital size and original (both years) vs. later (2nd year only) participation were examined and smaller hospitals who participated later performed better.
Hendriks, 2009[69]	To determine if managed competition and public reporting of quality information is associated with quality improvement in health plans.	National health plans; Health plan; Netherlands	Dutch Health Plans, and Health Plans on a National Level; Random sample of health Plan Members; CQI-based on CAHPS;	Observational, time series, no comparison group	3;1	Plans improved in some domains (health plan information and transparency of copayment, conduct of employees, and general rating and requirements, but not others(access to call center, getting needed help from call center and reimbursement of claims) from 2005 to 2008. Identification of selected domains as areas in need of improvement did not seem to affect whether there was improvement or not.
Kim, 2005[67]	To assess the impact of public release of hospital caesarean rates.	Caesarean Section Rates; Hospital; South Korea	263 hospitals	Observational, time series, no comparison group	2;1	Caesarean rates were 43.0% in 1999. Hospital data for 1999 were published in 2000 and rates declined to 38.6% in 2000 and 39.6% in 2001, which are lower than predicted based on rates for 1985 to 1999 and the first years with any decline. Multiple regression results found that hospitals with higher with higher baseline caesarean rates and higher volume were more likely to decline, while market share and financial incentives were not significantly associated with decline in rates.

Design ratings: 4 stars indicate a strong study design rating; while 1 star indicates a weaker study design rating.
Global ratings: 3 indicates great weight in the stratum's body of evidence; and 1 indicates little weight.

APPENDIX F. CRITERIA USED IN QUALITY ASSESSMENT

Fung and Colleagues' Grading Criteria for Included Studies

Study design ratings:

4 stars indicate a randomized trial or experimental trial;

3 stars indicate a controlled trial, pre-post trial with control (controlled before-after trial);

2 stars indicate a pre-post without control, observational cohort study without multivariable adjustment, cross-sectional study without multivariable adjustment, analysis of time trends without control, or well-designed qualitative study; and

1 star indicates a case series, other qualitative study, or survey (descriptive) study.

Global ratings:

3 indicates great weight in the stratum's body of evidence;

2 indicates moderate weight; and

1 indicates little weight.

AMSTAR Grading Criteria for Systematic Reviews

1. Was an 'a priori' design provided? The research question and inclusion criteria should be established before the conduct of the review.	☐ Yes ☐ No ☐ Can't answer ☐ Not applicable
2. Was there duplicate study selection and data extraction? There should be at least two independent data extractors and a consensus procedure for disagreements should be in place.	☐ Yes ☐ No ☐ Can't answer ☐ Not applicable
3. Was a comprehensive literature search performed? At least two electronic sources should be searched. The report must include years and databases used (e.g. Central, EMBASE, and MEDLINE). Key words and/or MESH terms must be stated and where feasible the search strategy should be provided. All searches should be supplemented by consulting current contents, reviews, textbooks, specialized registers, or experts in the particular field of study, and by reviewing the references in the studies found.	☐ Yes ☐ No ☐ Can't answer ☐ Not applicable
4. Was the status of publication (i.e. grey literature) used as an inclusion criterion? The authors should state that they searched for reports regardless of their publication type. The authors should state whether or not they excluded any reports (from the systematic review), based on their publication status, language etc.	☐ Yes ☐ No ☐ Can't answer ☐ Not applicable

5. Was a list of studies (included and excluded) provided?
A list of included and excluded studies should be provided.

☐ Yes
☐ No
☐ Can't answer
☐ Not applicable

6. Were the characteristics of the included studies provided?
In an aggregated form such as a table, data from the original studies should be provided on the participants, interventions and outcomes. The ranges of characteristics in all the studies analyzed e.g. age, race, sex, relevant socioeconomic data, disease status, duration, severity, or other diseases should be reported.

☐ Yes
☐ No
☐ Can't answer
☐ Not applicable

7. Was the scientific quality of the included studies assessed and documented?
'A priori' methods of assessment should be provided (e.g., for effectiveness studies if the author(s) chose to include only randomized, double-blind, placebo controlled studies, or allocation concealment as inclusion criteria); for other types of studies alternative items will be relevant.

☐ Yes
☐ No
☐ Can't answer
☐ Not applicable

8. Was the scientific quality of the included studies used appropriately in formulating conclusions?
The results of the methodological rigor and scientific quality should be considered in the analysis and the conclusions of the review, and explicitly stated in formulating recommendations.

☐ Yes
☐ No
☐ Can't answer
☐ Not applicable

9. Were the methods used to combine the findings of studies appropriate?
For the pooled results, a test should be done to ensure the studies were combinable, to assess their homogeneity (i.e. Chi-squared test for homogeneity, I^2). If heterogeneity exists a random effects model should be used and/or the clinical appropriateness of combining should be taken into consideration (i.e. is it sensible to combine?).

☐ Yes
☐ No
☐ Can't answer
☐ Not applicable

10. Was the likelihood of publication bias assessed?
An assessment of publication bias should include a combination of graphical aids (e.g., funnel plot, other available tests) and/or statistical tests (e.g., Egger regression test).

☐ Yes
☐ No
☐ Can't answer
☐ Not applicable

11. Was the conflict of interest stated?
Potential sources of support should be clearly acknowledged in both the systematic review and the included studies.

☐ Yes
☐ No
☐ Can't answer
☐ Not applicable

APPENDIX G. PEER REVIEW COMMENTS/AUTHOR RESPONSES

Peer Review Comments	Comment	Response
Scope	Thought the scope was too small. The literature in this area is pretty scant and did not need an ESP to tell us that. Would have expanded review to no just patients but organizations, VSO, other health care systems and other federal agencies	The scope was provided to us by the co-sponsor and is not something we can choose now.
	On pages 17 through 19 two long numbered lists are provided and referenced, but it's not clear if the entire lists are quoted verbatim from the original source. (This should be made clear if it is verbatim.)	These are not quoted verbatim, but rather summarized from the original report, which we now indicate.
	This is a superb and comprehensive review, but may short-change both public reporting and the VA, at least according to one authoritative published opinion. Lucian Leape recently concluded that public reporting was "So far, the most powerful method for reducing preventable injuries", and he went on to cite the VA's own NISQUIP program as the most shining example. (Transparency and public reporting are essential for a safe health care system. LL Leape. The Commonwealth Fund Publication 1381, Vol 4: "Perspectives on Health Reform". March 2010. Accepting that data showing that public reporting improves safety may not yet be strong, Leape's comments point out that this approach seems at least to have more potential than many of the alternatives (regulation, alignment of incentives, accreditation). I'd like to see this perspective mentioned in the discussion. I'd also like to see a brief data summary regarding studies that have looked at VA programs specifically.	This comment quotes Lucian Leape as stating public reporting is a "powerful method for reducing preventative injuries." We would agree that public reporting consistently influences providers to meet the criteria being reported. However NSQUIP cannot be used as an example, since NSQUIP is not publicly reported, at least not at the time of the studies documenting improvements due to NSQUIP.
	2nd paragraph, sentence beginning "Public reporting also…may only be known by providers" – awkward sentence	We have rewritten for clarity.
	2nd full paragraph re: hospitals in South Korea – unclear why data from non-English speaking country was included for this key question but not others.	We restricted KQ 1&2 to English speaking countries only since we judged that the context of the country mattered for questions about "how to most effectively display information" and "how do patients prefer to receive this information?" In other words, we thought data about how patients in non-English speaking countries such as Korea and the Netherlands would have limited relevance to the US. However, for KQ 3&4, about what effects public reporting has, we did not judge country context to be as important and therefore included studies from other countries.
	P. 26, 3rd full paragraph, last sentence – should be "difference was no longer significant" rather than "difference was no long significant". P. 26, 4th full paragraph, 1st sentence – should end with "selection of patients for procedures" instead of "patient". P. 29, Key Questions 1 and 2, last sentence – "assess" is misspelled.	Typo's are corrected

Peer Review Comments	Comment	Response
	P. 30, Acceptability of Findings to the VA Population, second sentence – Would suggest adding: "It is not clear whether public reporting would stimulate further changes in a system such as VA with a robust quality assessment and feedback system already in place." General comment – "Veteran" is sometimes capitalized in document and sometimes lowercase.	Text has been added.
	Methods: the discussion about excluding Fung articles, then adding them in, is confusing. Exclusion criteria should only focus on what is fully excluded from the synthesis.	This section has been updated for clarity.
	Of the 11 articles "rejected" because they focused onn individual providers, were there any global insights that impact questions 2 or 3? Are the trends/insights any different from those for hospitals/facilities?	We did not look into detail at the studies on individual providers. The Fung review did include such studies and concluded that in the few studies found results were mixed in the effect on selection of provider and un-clinical outcomes and unintended consequences; no studies were identified as quality improvement activities (11 studies were identified for hospitals).
	Add a section called Recommendations for VA. The section on applicability to the VA population does not get at issues specific to operations/implementation of public reporting of VA data. The Transparency initiative, for example, would benefit from learning more about Aligning Forces for Quality and their experience with providing community-level data to the public.	"Recommendations for VA" is not a heading in our report template. Rather our report provides evidence for a VA policymaker to make recommendations.
	Seems like a tepid conclusion in light of the actual studies. It seems like there is very little evidence that patients and families use reports. Any impact on market share or volume may, in fact, involve decisions made by payers, or the influence of other factors (like loss of accreditation, program closures, etc).	We agree that there is very little evidence that patients and families use reports. We think our existing statement that use is "moderate at best" accurately conveys this.

Peer Review Comments	Comment	Response
Scope	Consumer vs. Patient. There is some variation in use of the term patient and consumer. Both terms are important, yet will have different conceptual views by readers. To address this issue, it might be valuable to have statements early in the document that patient is meant to convey the Veteran and primary target of VA-related public data, and that consumer is a commonly-used term in discussion about public reporting of data. In general, for the purposes of the report, consider them interchangeable (keep in mind that consumer can include family members and informal caregivers, so is a broader and more inclusive term). Then pick one and use that for the rest of the report.	We have added these terms to the report.
	Definition of Provider. There are several uses of the term "provider" – from an individual doctor or clinician, to a hospital or clinic. This will be confusing for readers. Suggest using the term provider to refer to clinicians, and facility/health care provider spelled out for the latter.	Definition of provider - We disagree with this distinction and use of "provider" in the broad sense, which can be an individual provider (authors of those are excluded from the report) and also hospitals and health plans.
	Topic development: is the Office of Quality and Performance a VA or VHA entity?	It is a VHA entity.
	What were the Fung criteria (could state them, rather than relegate to Appendix).	Language has been modified.
	Literature flow: match the numbers in the narrative with the numbers in the diagram (3 or 6 studies from content experts??)	Numbers are now in agreement.
	Discussion about prior reviews is under Literature Flow. Consider a separate heading, such as Prior Review.	We have added this subheading.
	Figure 2: what do circles numbered 1 and 2 represent? The "one mention" and "two mentions" must be the explanation…but it's not immediately clear to the reader.	We have revised the legend for clarity.
	Key Question #1: why non-U.S. studies taken out? The comment about "particularly sensitive to context" makes the assumption that a person in Germany who gets health data is very different than a person in New York.	The cultural context here is around consumerism. The USA is considered a consumerist society, whereas all European countries have not been, although are becoming more so in the past 10 years.
	Key Question #2: maybe I missed this, but I didn't see much discussion about how patients want to receive or access this information…	This section included all the data and recommendations that were in the Hibbard & Sofaer and the RWJ reports, there is nothing more about this topic that we can include.
	Key Question #3, evidence from systematic review by Fung: Paragraph about the two pathways, and "change pathway" is confusing.	We have included a figure to better illustrate this.
	Impact on Clinical Outcomes: prior discussion excluded non-U.S. studies, and this section discusses S. Korean and Dutch studies; this is confusing (see #12 – consider all non-U.S. studies	We have now excluded non-US studies. Still need to check with AT.

Peer Review Comments	Comment	Response
Scope	Interesting items in Limitations discussion – why was the CHQC program abandoned? Why was the CHOP report not part of this review (only because it wasn't in a peer review journal?)	We did not know why the CHOP was abandoned, that was not in the scope. We have added the newer CHOP report as part of our revision to add relevant evidence identified via internet searches.
	Future research. Given the results of the report, there seem to be more research questions than those proposed. Was there any data about how consumers want to receive/access data? This is an important question that could be study variations in how the data is displayed is important, as well as credibility of the data, trust in the "deliverer" of the data (e.g. government). There are studies on numeracy and literacy and how to present data, although not specifically on publically reported data.	We have added this to the search question.
Search Related	Since there was very little in national work might have been interesting to also look at web sites and high quality blogs? Understand peer review is the best but if the data is not there need to look other places	This is a good suggestion and we have now incorporated a web search into the report. We added the Google search.
	Need large scope of review, maybe look more at social media and web info and not just published standard journals	
	If I were responsible for it the main thing I would want checked is the Google search mentioned above to see if the first few dozen "hits" identify any studies that should be added.	
	On page 30 the authors write that "public reporting of quality information" produces over 19,000,000 hits, but when the text is in quotes, it actually results in only 18,100 hits, and when the word "healthcare" is added separately to the search, then the number drops to 17,500, which is still a high number – but the first page of links look highly relevant to the study. Since I don't know which studies were excluded in Figure 1 there's no way to tell that the 22 new studies included in the report are the complete set of useful studies.	We have now incorporated a web search, but limited to the top 30 hits.
Database	The search methodology is described only briefly and incompletely. The methods say that the literature search was done "using standard search terms" and Appendix A, which is cited as the place to look for clarification, lists only a few author searches. This report would benefit from a comprehensive description of the search strategy, so that it can be checked and repeated in the future. If the exact terms were used as in the Fung report, that should be stated, or how the terms here differed.	Appendix A lists all the search terms and databases searched.
	Search strategy does not include search terms (would be helpful to see).	
	No terms for search presented (maybe this will be an appendix?)	The research terms and databases are in the appendix.

Peer Review Comments	Comment	Response
Nursing Home	Given the VA's provision of nursing home care, it would be preferable to have include nursing home care.	
	The objectives, scope, and methods for this review are clearly described, but I am not certain why the review excluded published information about public reporting of nursing homes, physicians or individual providers. Certainly, the VA statement of transparency does not preclude this, and while present plans have implemented publication of facility level quality information there is great interest and expectancies that the transparency will spread. The review would have far more useful if these areas were INCLUDED (since they represent future needs rather than retrospective) E.G. Having put up the website, now we pay a reviewer to identify how we should have done it (better late than never) , failure to include provider and nursing homes means we will always be chasing our tails.	Nursing homes and individual providers were not included in our scope as provided to us by central office.
	Study Selection #2, "nursing homes" – Since VA provides nursing home care, I would have liked to see this included	Nursing homes were not included in the scope provided to us.
	Scope is reasonably presented; however, the rationale for not including nursing homes and individual providers makes no sense. The key questions are not VA-specific, and if there is important information about the display of information or consumer use of information in decision-making, it would be of value here.	Nursing homes and individual providers were not included in our scope as provided to us by central office.
	Do any of the studies mention how hospital staff used the reports? Perhaps "internal transparency" can motivate quality improvement as much as external reporting. (Shame being, perhaps, an even greater motivator than money).	We did not look at "internal transparency" or reporting back to providers but not the public. The one study that directly assessed this question reported more quality improvement activity with public reporting.
Nursing Home	It is worth asking the question "what is missing". For instance, pure public reporting, without any other organized effort to address poor performance or ensure accountability, may simply be "information noise". On the other hand, if poor performers faced loss of accreditation, loss of business, or other penalties, they may be more likely to take action. It would be useful to know if any of the studies combined such managerial interventions with public reporting.	We did not assess the existence of managerial interventions, but think those can be assumed to exist, since without them plan and facility performance would be unlikely to change.
	Study selection: Need better rationale than "VA public reporting for facilities" for not including individual provider and nursing home data studies. The key questions are not VA specific, so it would be ideal to add these in.	The scope was given to us by central office and this is the rational they gave us.

Peer Review Comments	Comment	Response
Recommendations	Not clear how cites 10-12, 14-15 fit into an evidence review with the stated inclusion criteria. These seem more like suggestions/recommendations from a non-systematic review and seem much different than studies such as cites 37-39, for example.	The article and RWJ reports on public reporting are included because they are recommendations from high profile organizations made by experts and based in the evidence that is available. It seemed to us that our report would seem incomplete if it were missing these two key reports.
	Can you be more precise how Hibbard and Sofaer arrived at their conclusions? It will be essential to know if these recommendations are based on "expert consensus" versus empirical evidence, and what exactly the nature of the evidence is (e.g., user acceptability testing – what types of users, how was testing done, etc)	The Hibbard and Sofaer reports are their recommendations, based on the available evidence, which was somewhat thin. Some of their evidence was usability testing. We judged the Hibbard & Sofaer and the RWJ recommendations to represent the best available blend of evidence and opinion.
	Key Question #1 and #2: this section is well written and quite interesting to read. However, it seems like a summary of global recommendations from a few specific papers (Hibbard; Mazor) and less like a synthesis of data. How were these recommendations developed? What type of research was conducted to support the variety of comments and suggestions? While the literature is not large, it might be valuable to provide example of studies behind the suggestions.	
Update Searches	Is it possible to do a quick check, using the same search terms, for any new articles published since January 2011?	We have preformed and update search though August 2011 and incorporated the one new study meeting the inclusion criteria (N=1).
	Some of the newer reporting systems, such as CMS' Hospital Compare and the RWJ AF4Q pilots, are relatively recent. Hence, my earlier comment that we conduct a "quick peek" at literature published since Jan 2011.	We have done an update search, however, the one study meeting inclusion criteria was not about Hospital Compare or RWJ AF4Q.
Evidence & Summary	Quality of Evidence: the title suggests quality of the studies ("quality of evidence"); narrative is about impact on quality improvement efforts.	The narrative is meant to explain why the quality of evidence for these studies is generally low, namely why one study did a direct comparison.
	It would be good to restate or list what the Key Questions are before addressing them.	We have now restated the key questions in the executive summary.
	Summary: Consider repeating the Questions above each summary.	We have added this.